MALIGNANT MELANOMA OF THE SKIN AND MUCOUS MEMBRANE

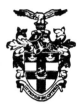

This book is dedicated to the patients and
staff of Sydney Hospital, in gratitude

MALIGNANT MELANOMA OF THE SKIN AND MUCOUS MEMBRANE

G. W. Milton, M.B.B.S.(Adel.), F.R.C.S., F.R.A.C.S.

Professor of Surgery, University of Sydney
Director of the Melanoma Unit, Sydney Hospital
Honorary Surgeon, Sydney Hospital
Visiting Professor in Surgery, Liverpool District Hospital

With chapters by

V. J. McGovern, M.D.(N.Z.), F.R.A.C.P., F.R.C.Path., F.R.C.P.A.

Director, Fairfax Institute of Pathology,
Royal Prince Alfred Hospital
President of the Royal College of Pathologists of Australia
Lecturer in Pathology, University of Sydney
Consultant to School of Public Health and Tropical Medicine,
University of Sydney

Martin G. Lewis, M.D., M.R.C.Path.(London)

Director, Cancer Research Unit,
McIntyre Medical Sciences Building, Montreal,
with the assistance of Geoffrey Rowden and
Terrence M. Phillips, McGill University Cancer Research Unit,
McIntyre Medical Sciences Building, Montreal

CHURCHILL LIVINGSTONE
Edinburgh London and New York 1977

CHURCHILL LIVINGSTONE
Medical Division of Longman Group Limited

Distributed in the United States of America by Longman
Inc., 19 West 44th Street, New York, N.Y. 10036 and by
associated companies, branches and representatives
throughout the world.

ISBN 0 443 01422 1

Library of Congress Cataloging in Publication Data
Milton, Gerald White, 1924–
    Malignant melanoma of the skin and mucous membrane.

    Includes index.
    1. Skin—Cancer. 2. Melanoma. 3. Mucous
membrane—Cancer. I. Title. [DNLM: 1. Melanoma.
2. Skin neoplasms. WR500 M662m]
RC280.S5M54   616.9′94′77   76-30318

Printed in Great Britain by
Butler & Tanner Ltd, Frome and London

Preface

Textbooks of medicine are often criticised because the authors are said to reproduce the mistakes of their predecessors, but they do have certain advantages. Professor J. Z. Young pointed out in his book *Introduction to the Study of Man* that at least they set out the opinion of the authors at any given time. The main tenet of this book has been that the authors describe to a very large degree their personal experience.

Over many years malignant melanoma has acquired a reputation of being virtually a death sentence, but in more recent times it is quite obvious that the disease is nowhere near as lethal as formerly supposed, especially if the conditions can be diagnosed and treated early. It is with this in mind that both the pathology and the clinical features of the disease are discussed in some detail, especially the problems relating to diagnosis. It may seem somewhat strange that lesions of the skin, which are the most superficial of all bodily ailments, are frequently not discussed from the point of view of their clinical history, and it is for this reason that some stress has been placed on the clinical history of malignant melanoma. The clinical history of this disease, both of the primary and of the metastases, is often characteristic. In addition the clinical aspects of this book are designed to help cope with some clinical problems that may be rare in the majority of surgical practices but are common in the practice of the Melanoma Unit at Sydney Hospital. The personal experience described in this book has been gained while working in the Department of Surgery at the University of Sydney and in the Sydney Hospital Melanoma Clinic. As far as possible in the text the sources of all references and ideas have been acknowledged, but in the course of many years' work it is sometimes difficult to remember the exact source of an idea or speculation; any omissions are inadvertent and any worker who feels slighted is asked please to accept our apologies.

The clinical aspects of this book have been very largely extracted from the Jacksonian Prize Essay of 1973. The sections on Pathology and that on Immunology and Immunotherapy have been written by men who have contributed a great deal in both these fields and I am very grateful to them for their contributions to this book.

A lifetime of experience is apt to build a large number of debts of gratitude, but to acknowledge them in detail would involve a considerable list. Throughout my time in the Department of Surgery in Sydney University, I have had much help from most members of the staff in all stages of this work and I am very grateful for it. Associate Professor W. H. McCarthy has given me invaluable assistance as my associate in the clinic over the past ten years. In the practice at Sydney Hospital it has been my great pleasure and privilege to work with many young people who have contributed a great deal to the book. I am reluctant to mention any by name in case inadvertently I omit someone who may be hurt by the omission. However, I cannot deny myself the pleasure of acknowledging Mrs M. Conroy for her loyal support and help over many years and for typing innumerable letters concerning the patients reported here. Mr G. Maxwell, Head Technician, who has been able to turn his hand to many aspects of administration, has helped in innumerable ways. I am also very grateful to Mrs S. Beamish, Mrs L. Ianello and Miss F. Bitter for their unstinting help in typing the manuscript through all its various revisions. The

Clinical Photographic Department of Sydney Hospital (Mr R. Money and Miss J. Stirling) have always been more than willing to help with their considerable skill with a camera, and the University Department of Illustration (Mr K. Clifford, Mr R. Scobie and Mr B. Bombell) have all helped me immensely. I am also very grateful to Dr V. J. McGovern and Dr Tania Jelihowsky at the Royal Prince Alfred Hospital, who in the early days of my interest in this subject were always willing to discuss cases and be helpful in every possible way. An old friend now deceased, Dr Jack Garvan, Director of the Pathology Department at St Vincent's Hospital, was also a constant source of friendly help.

During the preparation of the manuscript I have been greatly helped by Margaret Power, librarian, Sydney Hospital, and by members of the Churchill Livingstone staff, and I am grateful to them.

A great deal of the research mentioned here has been supported by three organisations, The New South Wales State Cancer Council, the Sydney University Research Fund and the Bill White Melanoma Research Fund. It is a particular pleasure for me to acknowledge the Bill White Melanoma Research Fund in a special way. It was a fund set up by the relatives and friends of a young man who died from malignant melanoma. Their resources to establish this fund were minimal but by a dint of great personal sacrifice and effort they have raised sufficient money to help the clinic in a large number of ways, and without their help a great deal of the work reported here would have been very difficult or even impossible to do.

Last, but by no means least, I can never fully repay all that I owe my wife and three children for their constant support, help and encouragement.

The study of malignant melanoma tends to become depressing and is a great drain on the emotional resources of those engaged in it. Throughout this work I have been sustained in a way that I would never have imagined possible by three groups of people: firstly, my family; secondly, the staff at Sydney Hospital; and thirdly the very real courage of a large number of patients whom it has been my privilege to look after.

1977   G. W. M.

Contents

1. Aetiology of Melanoma; Classification and Histological Reporting; Spontaneous Regression; Frozen Section Diagnosis

V. J. McGovern

AETIOLOGY OF MELANOMA

In studying the aetiology of melanoma there is a tendency to place too much emphasis on the incidence in areas such as Queensland (Beardmore, 1972) where a susceptible population is reacting almost to its maximal ability, whereas a clearer insight into some of the underlying factors may be more readily ascertainable from a study of the incidence in countries such as Norway (Magnus, 1973), Sweden (Lee and Issenberg, 1972), Britain (Lee and Carter, 1970) or Israel (Movshovitz and Modan, 1973) where melanoma occurs much less commonly.

Melanoma is increasing in its incidence amongst white races, not only in areas of high incidence such as Queensland where the rate has quadrupled in 30 years (Beardmore, 1972), but also in areas such as Norway (Magnus, 1973), Britain (Lee and Carter, 1970), the United States (Lee, 1973) and Canada (Elwood and Lee, 1974) in which the incidences have doubled since the Second World War. The mortality has increased correspondingly with a sharp rise in those aged less than 45 years (Lee, 1973). This increased incidence has not occurred amongst other skin cancers, and in some countries the death rate from these has actually declined (Lee and Issenberg, 1972).

It is clear that the problem of aetiology is a complicated one and that there are both genetic and environmental aspects to be considered.

First of all it is necessary to consider the part played by pigmented naevi in the development of melanoma. Naevi are very common and though the clinical evidence suggests that most melanomas commence in naevi, only a very small fraction of the total number of moles in the population become malignant.

The relationship between naevi and melanoma

Until 1892 when Jonathan Hutchinson described the lesion we now know as Hutchinson's melanotic freckle, it was believed that all melanomas arose in pre-existent naevi (Paget, 1864). The proportion that commences in naevi cannot be determined with accuracy but nearly two-thirds of patients state that there had been a pre-existent pigmented lesion and the majority of these noted that there had been a recent change in the lesion (Milton, 1972).

When a melanoma commences in a junction naevus, the histological pattern of the naevus is usually lost, and only in occasional cases does the typical pattern of a junction naevus persist at the edge of the lesion. However, in about 25 per cent of melanomas there is an accompanying intradermal naevus, which presupposes that there had been a compound naevus and that the melanoma had arisen in its junctional component (McGovern, 1970). The circumstantial evidence, then, supports the view that most melanomas develop in pre-existent naevi.

Generally naevi are much more common in the white than in the black races, although surprisingly, according to a survey by Pack, Davis and Oppenheim (1963), Filipinos, Japanese and Maoris have more pigmented naevi than white Americans, who averaged 14 per person. The average number of naevi amongst Sydney University students is 16 (unpublished data). Naevi are most common in the face and neck and on the back. However, these are not necessarily the commonest sites of melanoma. In the state of Connecticut where melanoma is an uncommon tumour, the commonest site in men is the head and neck while the leg is the most common site in women (Clark and MacDonald, 1953). In Queensland melanoma is a common neoplasm; the commonest site of melanoma in men is the trunk, but the leg is still the commonest site for women (Beardmore, 1972). Though the head and neck is not the most frequent site in Queensland the percentage of melanomas in that site increases with age.

These facts indicate that the development of a melanoma depends upon a number of aetiological factors and not only the presence of a junction naevus.

Associated intradermal naevi can be demonstrated histologically in about one-quarter of all melanomas (McGovern, 1970), suggesting that in these cases the tumour commenced in a compound naevus. Since two-thirds of patients state that their melanoma commenced in a pre-existent pigmented lesion (Milton, 1972), the presumption is that the difference between this figure and the number of naevi shown histologically (more than 40 per cent) is made up of melanomas commencing in junctional naevi, the remaining one-third arising *de novo*.

There is one variety of naevus, however, in which there is a greatly augmented malignant potential. This is the giant congenital naevi, which frequently has a garment distribution and frequently has a number of smaller lesions of similar type scattered over the body. They are usually a mixture of intradermal and compound naevi and scattered smaller lesions, especially in children, which may be junctional naevi. Blue naevi may be present also. When malignancy supervenes, it is not always possible to find the exact site of the primary growth and in some cases it seems to have commenced in the blue naevus component. Greeley, Middleton and Curtin (1965) observed the development of malignancy in 10 of 56 cases they collected over a period of 25 years, and collected 20 other examples from the literature of melanoma arising in giant naevi. Reed *et al.* (1965) collected 55 examples of giant congenital naevi in 17 of which there was malignant

melanoma. The exact incidence of melanoma arising in giant naevi is not known. It is certainly greater than it is for ordinary non-congenital naevi, and in different series has varied from 1·8 to 13·0 per cent.

Because giant pigmented naevi have a greater tendency to malignancy than non-congenital naevi, Mark *et al.* (1973) have commenced a study of small congenital naevi in order to find out whether or not these, too, have a heightened malignancy potentiality. So far the question remains unanswered.

If the inhabitants of Queensland have the same number of moles as Sydney University students then it can be calculated that with an incidence of 16 melanomas per 100 000 of population, the melanoma rate in that State is 1 per 100 000 pigmented naevi. In other States where the incidence of melanoma is lower the number of moles undergoing malignant transformation would be even fewer.

Racial factors

Melanoma is a rare neoplasm in the dark-skinned races. This feature is strikingly illustrated in the figures from South Africa quoted by Oettle (1966) in which he compared the death rates of the three groups, Whites, Coloureds and Asians. The Coloureds are a mulatto race descended from Malays and Hottentots admixed with white and to some extent Bantu. The Asians are mainly Indian. The death rate for melanoma amongst Whites was more than twice that of Coloureds, while the death rate amongst Asians was extremely low.

Similarly the incidence of melanoma amongst Indians in India (Sampat and Sirsat, 1966), Blacks in the United States (MacDonald, 1959), Indonesians (Pringgoutoma and Pringgoutoma, 1963), Japanese (Mori, 1973) and New Guineans (Reay-Young and Wilkey, 1974) and other dark-skinned races are low compared with the incidence in white-skinned races. Nevertheless, in areas of low incidence, melanoma amongst dark-skinned persons may occur as commonly as amongst white-skinned persons, though the site-distribution may be different. The incidence in Uganda (Lewis, 1967) for instance, varies between 1·4 and 3·8 per 100 000. Compared with England and Wales (The Registrar General's Statistical Review, 1965) where the rate is 1·4 for men and 2·3 for women per 100 000, this seems high. However, there is a difference in site-incidence: as in all dark-skinned races the predominant site is the foot.

In her study of melanoma in Texas, Eleanor MacDonald (1959) found that the annual incidence amongst Blacks was 1·28 per 100 000 and 1·2 per 100 000 amongst Latin Americans and Anglo-Americans. Though the incidence of melanoma was higher than one would have expected in Blacks, there was a fundamental difference in site-distribution between Blacks on the one hand and Latin Americans and Anglo-Americans on the other. Amongst Texan Blacks, the foot was the commonest site. Amongst Latin Americans the incidences of melanoma in the head and neck, the trunk, the upper extremity and the lower extremity were similar. In Texan Anglo-Americans the head and neck was the principal site.

It is clear that although pigment protects, melanoma still occurs in dark-skinned races. The site-incidences, however, are different from those in white races. Amongst these people there is a proportionately higher incidence in the sole of the foot and in the mucosae. Amongst 119 melanomas reported by Sampat and Sirsat (1966) in India, for example, 41 were mucosal, and of the 78 cutaneous melanomas 42 occurred in the foot. Similarly in other dark-skinned peoples, the sole of the foot is the commonest site. It seems an inescapable conclusion that the relative susceptibility of the sole of the foot and the mucosae in these races is associated with lack of pigment in those sites rather than a particular racial susceptibility.

However, even amongst the white races there are different degrees of susceptibility, the most notable being the susceptibility of Swedes and Norwegians (The Registrar General's Statistical Review, 1965) to the development of melanoma and of persons of Celtic descent to the development of skin cancer of all types including melanoma (Lane Brown et al., 1971; Lane Brown and Lelia, 1973).

In Sweden and Norway the incidences of melanoma are higher than in England and Wales (The Registrar General's Statistical Review, 1965) although those countries are situated at a higher latitude. The incidence in England and Wales for the years 1962–1965 was 1·4 per 100 000 for men and 2·4 for women while in Sweden in the same period the incidence was 3·9 per 100 000 for men and 4·2 for women (Lee and Issenberg, 1972). The incidence in Norway is similar to that in Sweden and in both the death rate is correspondingly higher than it is in England and Wales (The Registrar General's Statistical Review, 1965).

Lane Brown et al. (1971) showed that in Sydney the incidence of melanoma as well as of other skin cancers in Celts is double that which would be expected from the proportion of Celts in the population. Similar results were obtained from a survey carried out in Boston (Lane Brown and Lelia, 1973).

From the foregoing brief discussion of racial susceptibility to the development of melanoma, the available evidence indicates that pigment protects and that in the dark-skinned races melanoma occurs relatively frequently in the lesser pigmented zones, such as the sole of the foot, and certain squamous mucosae, such as that of the oral cavity, the anorectal mucosa, the vagina, the nasal mucosa and penis. Why this should be so is unexplained.

Sunlight as a cause of melanoma

The possibility that solar radiation played a part in the aetiology of melanoma was first suggested by McGovern (1952). He noted that amongst patients of Royal Prince Alfred Hospital, the head and neck in both men and women and the legs in women were the most commonly affected sites. This stimulated the work of Lancaster (1956), who then showed that the death rate, and presumably the incidence of melanoma, increased with proximity to the equator. This relationship of latitude with melanoma pertains in the Northern (Magnus, 1973; Bodenham, 1968; Elwood *et al.*, 1974; MacDonald, Wolf and Johnson, 1970) as well as in the Southern Hemisphere. In Australia the death rate from melanoma for the years 1961 to 1970 ranges from 25 per 100 000 in Victoria, which is the State farthest from the equator, to 47 per 100 000 in Queensland, which is partly within the tropics (Beardmore, 1972). This trend can be observed even in countries with a lower incidence of melanoma, as in Norway (Magnus, 1973) where melanoma is three times as common in the south as in the north. This north–south gradient in the Northern Hemisphere is also present in Britain (Bodenham, 1968), Canada (Elwood and Lee, 1974) and the United States (MacDonald *et al.*, 1970; Lee, 1972).

In addition to the effect of latitude or residence on the incidence of melanoma, the duration of residence in a place with much sunshine is also of importance. This is well illustrated by the incidence of melanoma in Israel. Movshovitz and Modan (1973) found that the incidence rate for melanoma was highest in native-born Israelis of European origin, intermediate in foreign-born Europeans who had had a long residence in Israel, and lower in recent European-born immigrants. The lowest rate was in Asian- and African-born immigrants.

However, though all the evidence links exposure to sunlight with the occurrence of melanoma, there are certain anomalies. In southern parts of Australia the exposed parts of the body, *viz.* the leg in the woman, the head and neck in the man and to a lesser extent in the woman, are the predominant sites for melanoma (Beardmore, 1972; McGovern, 1970; McGovern, 1966; Central Cancer Registry, Report No. 2, 1962; Lee, 1970). Closer to the equator where the incidence is higher, as in Queensland, there is an increased incidence in less exposed sites such as the trunk in both sexes (Beardmore, 1972). Furthermore the relative rates between men and women for the legs which are normally covered in men and exposed in women are similar in Queensland (Beardmore, 1972) where the incidence of melanoma is very high, and in New South Wales where the occurrence of melanoma is much lower (McGovern, 1970). One would have expected an increase in the proportion of women to men with melanoma of the leg in Queensland, but this is not so.

These anomalous facts led to the postulate that as well as having a direct effect upon cutaneous melanocytes, ultraviolet light produces in the skin a factor which can enter the bloodstream and act upon susceptible melanocytes in other parts of the body (Lee and Merrill, 1970). This concept is supported by the studies of Black and Lo (1971), who found that ultraviolet irradiation of human skin produced photo-oxidation products of cholesterol which were carcinogenic for rats and mice. If this pertains in the development of melanoma, the increasing incidence of this tumour would mean that there is an increasing concentration in the skin of some substance that can be converted into a carcinogen by solar radiation, perhaps some dietary substance that is becoming more commonly used, or some other environmental factor that is increasing in amounts or intensity.

While the above arguments may have some validity, it is more probable that the increased incidence of melanoma amongst white races living in latitudes of intense sunshine is a direct effect of solar exposure.

A paradoxical situation arises out of the high incidence of melanoma in the trunk, particularly the back, because the trunk is usually a covered area of the body. This, up to a point, is true, but the covering is often a transparent material that permits the passage of ultraviolet light. Many fair people become sunburned through their light shirts or blouses. Examination of the plotted site-incidence of melanoma shows that areas covered with a double layer of clothing and hence non-transparent are affected in a random way. Melanoma is not common in the skin of the female breast which normally is protected by a brassière, nor in the genital and buttock regions which are also normally covered by non-transparent clothing. In the more temperate zones of Australia, the head and neck in both sexes together with the leg of the female are the commonest sites of melanoma (Beardmore, 1972; McGovern, 1970; McGovern, 1966; Central Cancer Registry, Report No. 2, 1962). These are exposed areas which are reacting almost to their maximum capacity in the production of melanoma. The back is less frequently exposed and the tendency is for melanoma to occur there in a random manner. In Queensland where light translucent clothing is the rule, the back is subjected to a greater dosage of ultraviolet light and can react maximally. The increase in melanoma of the back would therefore be proportionately much greater than in the head and neck regions.

Dr T. B. Fitzpatrick of Boston has been reiterating for more than 10 years that apparently non-exposed areas of skin may still be receiving injurious amounts of ultraviolet light through the clothing, and therefore each patient has to be individually assessed according to his or her dress habits.

One of the arguments advanced against sunlight as a cause of melanoma is that the site-incidences of basal cell carcinoma and squamous cell carcinoma of the skin are unrelated to the site-incidences of melanoma.

Basal and squamous cell carcinomas occur most frequently in exposed skin, and the incidence is higher in Queensland where solar exposure is greater than in the southern states of Australia where the exposure is less. The increased incidence is confined to the exposed parts of the body, and unlike melanoma the unexposed parts are for the most part unaffected (Gordon, Silverstone and Smithurst, 1972).

The fact that squamous cell carcinoma and basal cell carcinoma do not occur with increased frequency in the same sites as melanoma in Queensland is not relevant since the cells giving rise to these tumours are developmentally different from the cells giving rise to melanoma. Squamous cell carcinoma and basal cell carcinomas for the most part arise in skin with severe solar damage. Melanomas, apart from those arising in Hutchinson's melanotic freckle, are associated with a much less severe degree of solar damage. From these considerations it seems likely that melanocytes are much more susceptible to the effects of solar irradiation than the other cells of the epidermis.

Mechanism of solar carcinogenesis

Ultraviolet light is the main source of stimulation of melanogenesis in human skin, but at the same time excessive solar radiation can have a deleterious effect. The cancer-producing segment of the spectrum lies between 290 nm and 320 nm and this also coincides with the erythemogenic portion of the spectrum. The cancer-producing effect of ultraviolet light is probably through the action of 'free radicals' (Norins, 1962; Pathak, 1966). Ultraviolet light has a high energy content and is capable of removing an electron from a susceptible molecule. Being left with an unpaired electron renders a molecule very reactive and it seems probable that such 'free radicals' cause the damage which results from excessive exposure to ultraviolet light. Some free radicals are destroyed by converting -SH compounds into disulphides while others are trapped by melanin (Norins, 1962). Any deficiency of melanin therefore is conducive to solar damage. Supporting this view is the finding by Pathak (1966) that free radicals are present in skin irradiated by light with a wavelength of 300 nm and that they were more prominent in unpigmented skin than in pigmented skin.

Each epidermal melanocyte yields its pigment granules to keratinocytes in close association with its dendritic processes. This group of keratinocytes together with its related melanocyte is sometimes designated the 'epidermal–melanin unit' (Fitzpatrick and Breathnach, 1963). Although the melanin is gradually degraded as it is carried towards the surface, there is sufficient in well-pigmented persons to protect the multiplying and therefore viable cells of the basal region of the epidermis. Amongst the cells protected by pigment in the overlying keratinocytes are the melanocytes.

Lancaster and Nelson (1957) demonstrated that those most commonly affected by melanoma in Australia were persons with fair skins who did not tan readily but who burned and freckled. These features have been noted in other parts of the world also.

Melanoma in albinos is rare and records can be found of only six cutaneous examples to date (Kennedy and Zelickson, 1963). In three of the six cases the melanoma commenced in a pre-existent naevus. The case of Kennedy and Zelickson (1963) was proved by the demonstration of premelanosomes by electron-microscopy.

Vitiligo is a common disorder, but though it may accompany melanoma I have not seen melanoma developing in a patch of vitiligo.

Abnormal responses to sunlight may be due to errors of metabolism, either inborn or acquired, the latter being due mainly to drugs and toxins.

Genetic sensitivity to sunlight is seen in xeroderma pigmentosum. In this condition solar keratoses, basal cell carcinomas and squamous cell carcinomas are common and death is usually due to dissemination of squamous cell carcinoma. In a few cases, however, melanoma, either melanotic or amelanotic, occurs. It is usually a highly malignant melanoma without any adjacent intra-epidermal component and may affect quite young children.

Many drugs cause photosensitivity but none has yet been demonstrated to have enhanced the carcinogenic action of ultraviolet light.

Familial aspects

The familial occurrence of cutaneous melanoma was first reported by Cawley in 1952. Since then there have been enough reported examples to establish the fact that there are certain families in which melanoma has occurred more frequently than can be attributed to chance. Anderson, Smith and McBride (1967) have documented the familial occurrence of melanoma in 22 kindreds, including one in which it occurred in a total of 15 individuals. In these 22 kindred, melanoma occurred in 67 individuals. They found that melanoma in this group occurred at an earlier age than that generally reported, i.e. occurring

at an average of $40{\cdot}7 \pm 1{\cdot}7$ years as opposed to $49{\cdot}0 \pm 0{\cdot}5$ years. The ages in this context are for patients at the M. D. Anderson Hospital, Houston, Texas; in countries where melanoma is a more common disease the average age at onset is lower than in countries where it is less common (McGovern, 1966).

Six (27 per cent) of the 22 propositi in the series of Anderson et al. (1967) had two or more melanomas which were histologically primary growths. Of the affected relatives three (21 per cent) had multiple primary tumours. There appears to be a definite proclivity for multiple primary lesions amongst patients with familial melanoma, and amongst the 85 patients recorded up to the time when Anderson et al. (1967) published their figures, there were 16 (19 per cent) with more than one primary tumour.

Allen and Spitz (1953) recorded 12 instances of multiple primary melanoma amongst their 337 cases (3·6 per cent) while Pack, Scharnagel and Hillyer (1952) found only 16 amongst 1250 (1·28 per cent).

In England, Peterson, Bodenham and Lloyd (1962) recorded an incidence of 2·3 per cent. In Queensland where every case was recorded there were 10 examples in 498 cases, an incidence of 2 per cent (Wallace and Exton, 1972). From these figures it is clear that melanoma patients are predisposed to the development of a second primary melanoma, and amongst patients with familial melanoma there is a still greater predisposition.

Anderson et al. (1967) found that multiple primary melanomas in their familial cases were most frequently found in the exposed parts of the body. In an unpublished series of 27 patients with multiple primary melanomas with no familial incidence Milton and McGovern did not find any site-predominance. This randomness indicates the probability of endogenous factors in causation.

From the study of Anderson et al. (1967) it seems clear that there is a genetic factor in familial melanoma. The number of relatives with melanoma in their series averaged 3·0. In fact eight of the 22 kindreds contained three or more affected relatives. With a population incidence of one melanoma per 100 000 in Texas, the probability of melanoma occurring in three members of a family is extremely remote and the probability of 28 patients with melanoma amongst 1000 patients purely on the basis of chance is likewise remote. For these reasons familial melanoma is regarded as hereditary melanoma.

Wallace and Exton (1972) in a meticulous and detailed study have shown that in Queensland, too, there is a heightened incidence of melanoma among the relatives of melanoma propositi, there being an incidence of 1·17 per cent among first-degree relatives of melanoma patients and of 5·6 per cent amongst the first-degree relatives in families where two cases had been recorded.

They demonstrated also that familial melanoma occurred most commonly amongst persons of Celtic origin, but there were no inherited features such as colour of the hair, eyes or skin or even in their reactivity to ultraviolet light, which differed in the group with familial melanoma from those with no family history of melanoma.

In contrast to the definite pattern of site-involvement by melanoma generally in Queensland, there was a random distribution of such involvement in inherited melanoma in keeping with its endogenous origins.

While the occurrence of melanoma in familial cases is clearly not sex-linked, the mode of inheritance is not clear.

In summary, patients with hereditary melanoma tend on this average to get melanoma at an earlier age than the general population and have a tendency to develop additional primary tumours.

Hormonal aspects

In many published series of melanoma there is a higher incidence in women than in men due to the larger numbers in the lower leg of women (Beardmore, 1972; McGovern, 1970; Lee, 1970; Peterson et al., 1962), but paradoxically the mortality rate is higher in men than in women (Beardmore, 1972; Lee, 1973; McGovern, 1970; Lee, 1970; Peterson et al.,

1962). The better survival rates in women have been said by some to pertain only in the child-bearing age. However, the figures from the Queensland Melanoma Project show that the death rate increases with age and that even in the postmenopausal decades the mortality for women is strikingly lower than that for men (Beardmore, 1972).

The fact that melanomas are more common after puberty than before is simply part of the phenomenon of increasing incidence of melanoma with age and not a result of puberty having an adverse effect upon junction naevi.

It used to be thought that pregnancy had an adverse effect upon survival from melanoma but this is now known not to be so (George, Fortner and Pack, 1960; White et al., 1961). George et al. (1960) found that in a series of 115 patients with melanoma diagnosed during pregnancy and compared with a similar group of non-pregnant patients the survival rates were identical. They thought, however, that the metastases were larger and blacker than in non-pregnant patients. This, of course, could be due to the augmented production of MSH elicited by the increased circulating oestrogens associated with the pregnant state (McGuiness, 1963).

The possibility that pregnancy can provoke the development of melanoma was investigated by Lee and Hill (1970). They analysed the deaths from melanoma in England and Wales for the years 1959–1967 according to marital status, because death certificates in England and Wales do not record pregnancy though they do record marital status. They found that the death rates of women with melanoma were the same in both the married and unmarried. The inference from this is that marriage and therefore pregnancy does not have any effect upon the incidence of melanoma.

There have been reports from time to time of spontaneous regression of melanoma with the termination of pregnancy (Boyd, 1966). The spontaneous regression of cutaneous melanoma, either partial or complete, is relatively common and occurs in both the pregnant and non-pregnant (McGovern, 1975). We have never seen the spontaneous regression of metastatic visceral melanoma on the termination of pregnancy.

We believe that there has been unnecessary apprehension about the possibility of pregnancy inducing melanoma or adversely affecting the outcome of an already existent melanoma.

Unresolved aetiological problems

Apart from the rare malignancy in a blue naevus there are three main histogenetic types of melanoma each with distinctive clinical and histological features (McGovern, 1970; Clark, 1967; McGovern *et al.*, 1973). These are melanoma arising in Hutchinson's melanotic freckle, melanoma with an adjacent intra-epidermal component of superficial spreading type, and melanoma with no adjacent intra-epidermal component. The reasons for the types of histogenetic development are obscure. They may be due in part to a balance between host resistance on the one hand and tumour invasiveness on the other. Melanoma arising in Hutchinson's melanotic freckle, however, is almost invariably associated with severe solar degeneration of the skin. Nevertheless, occasional examples of Hutchinson's melanotic freckle are found in persons of fair complexion in their twenties who have comparatively little solar degeneration of the skin. Then again, not every person with severe solar degeneration of the skin develops Hutchinson's melanotic freckle. From these considerations it may be inferred that there are two factors involved, *viz.* individual susceptibility and a critical accumulation of solar radiation, each of these two factors being variable.

At the other end of the spectrum is melanoma arising in the sole of the foot or in the various mucosae of dark-skinned persons in which solar radiation could not have played any part. For these an endogenous cause must be postulated.

There is currently an increase in the incidence of melanoma in various parts of the world as well as in Australia. This raises the question that perhaps some agent in the environment is rendering some persons more susceptible to solar radiation. Sunlight seems to be the most important aetiological agent in the development of melanoma, but there are many other factors which enhance or modify susceptibility, of which the most important are race, degree of cutaneous pigmentation, geographical latitude, and ability to tan on exposure to sunlight.

THE CLASSIFICATION AND HISTOLOGICAL REPORTING OF MELANOMA

Histogenetic types of melanoma

In 1864 Sir James Paget said that it was well known that cancer could arise in or under a mole. However, not until 1892 when Jonathan Hutchinson described the lesion we now call Hutchinson's melanotic freckle was it realised that pigmented lesions could appear in adult life which could give rise to melanoma. Dubreuilh (1912), who had followed the same line of thought as Hutchinson, pointed out that melanoma could arise *ab initio* in previously blemish-free skin. Hutchinson called his lesion *senile freckle* because it occurred in the sun-damaged skin of elderly people, the commonest site being the malar region and temple. In 1894, when Hutchinson published the first example of melanoma arising in a *senile freckle*, he altered the name to *lentigo-melanosis* and included in this category macular pigmented lesions on non-exposed parts of the body, the prepuce for example, which he believed to be capable of malignant transformation. Dubreuilh acted similarly. He did not like the name *senile freckle* and changed the name to *mélanose circonscrite précancéreuse*, a term which has entered the dermatological vocabulary as *melanosis circumscripta praecancerosa* of Dubreuilh, and throughout the world people have included under the one category the lesions of Hutchinson's melanotic freckle and flat pigmented lesions on the covered parts of the body. Dubreuilh noted that these two types of lesion behaved differently in that a nodule of recognisable invasive melanoma arising in *melanosis circumscripta praecancerosa* on the covered parts of the body such as the leg had a much worse prognosis than an invasive nodule arising in *melanosis circumscripta praecancerosa* in the sun-damaged skin of the face. In an attempt to clarify the situation a group of Australian pathologists (Committee of Australian Pathologists, 1967) decided that *melanosis circumscripta praecancerosa* should be divided into two groups, namely *Hutchinson's melanotic freckle* and *premalignant melanosis*. Around about the same time Clark (1967) divided *melanosis circumscripta praecancerosa* into *lentigo maligna* (*Hutchinson's melanotic freckle*) and *superficial spreading melanoma*. Melanoma without any spreading pigmentation was called nodular melanoma by Clark. Clark *et al.* (1969) found that each of these three types of melanoma had a different prognosis; that nodular melanoma had the worst prognosis; and melanoma arising in Hutchinson's melanotic freckle (*lentigo maligna*) had the best prognosis. In Australia also it was found that these three groups had different prognoses.

In 1972 at the time of the UICC Cancer Congress in Sydney on the subject of Melanoma and Skin Cancer, a number of pathologists met to devise a suitable classification for the reporting of melanoma. Their classification (McGovern *et al.*, 1973) was:

1. Invasive malignant melanoma with an adjacent intra-epidermal component of Hutchinson's melanotic freckle type.

2. Invasive malignant melanoma with an adjacent intra-epidermal component of superficial spreading type.

3. Invasive malignant melanoma with an adjacent intra-epidermal component of unclassifiable type.

4. Invasive malignant melanoma without an adjacent intra-epidermal component.

Hutchinson's melanotic freckle (Fig. 1.1)

Hutchinson's melanotic freckle occurs most commonly in the malar region and often involves the lower eyelid. It is an irregular macular lesion varying in colour between brown and

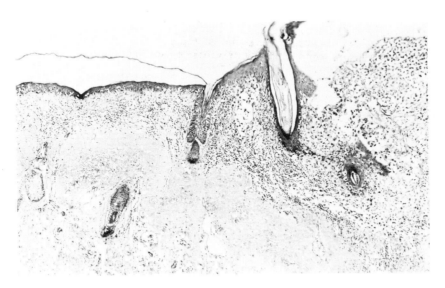

Fig. 1.1 A female aged 47 years with a Hutchinson's melanotic freckle of the cheek in which nodules had appeared. The photomicrographs illustrate the essential features of Hutchinson's melanotic freckle.

a. Low power view showing a portion of invasive melanoma with atrophic epidermis and hair follicles, in which the basal melanocytes have proliferated. There is a lymphocytic infiltrate beneath the melanoma and also beneath the Hutchinson's freckle. There is severe solar degeneration of the dermis. H & E × 48.

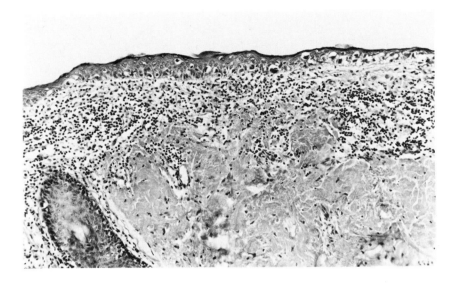

Fig. 1.1   b. There is proliferation of melanocytes with very irregular nuclei. The melanocytes are mainly in the basal region. There is severe solar degeneration of the dermis and a lymphocytic infiltrate in the upper dermis. H & E × 120.

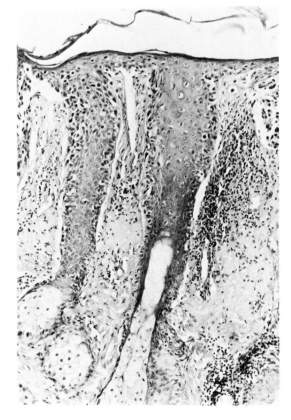

c. This photomicrograph illustrates the hair follicle involvement in Hutchinson's melanotic freckle. H & E × 120.

black. It often has paler areas which represent areas of spontaneous regression. Hutchinson noted that the lesion had a tendency to advance and recede like an infective process, and indeed the lesion has been known to disappear completely only to recur again after a period of months or years. Before the development of invasive nodules, the lesion is impalpable. Eventually after a period averaging 10 to 15 years and sometimes much longer one or more nodules of invasive melanoma appear in the lesion. These nodules may be amelanotic as in the case described by Hutchinson (1894). Hutchinson's melanotic freckle enlarges slowly and by the time it develops a nodule of melanoma it may measure several centimetres across. It is not uncommon to see a Hutchinson's melanotic freckle measuring up to 6 or 8 cm in its longest extent. Nevertheless, a nodule of melanoma can arise in a Hutchinson's melanotic freckle that is quite small, no more than 1 to 2 cm in extent.

The sites where this lesion is found are those which receive the maximum amount of solar irradiation, particularly the malar regions and the temples, but they also occur in other areas of the face. They can occur on the neck, both posteriorly and anteriorly, and they have been observed on the backs of hands and wrists. In all these sites there is severe solar degeneration of the skin, usually with atrophy of appendages.

Microscopic appearances

Microscopically Hutchinson's melanotic freckle is just as distinctive as it is clinically. The typical histological features are best seen in a lesion that has not yet developed an invasive melanoma, or if there is a melanoma present, at the edge of the spreading macular pigmentation. There one finds that the melanocytes in the basal layer of the epidermis are large and round with irregular nuclei, and these atypical melanocytes extend down the outer root sheath of the hair follicles (Fig. 1.1). Sometimes it is difficult to decide whether or not there is actual increase in numbers of melanocytes in the early lesion. As the melanocytes become more numerous and are in contact with each other they tend to palisade. Eventually small clusters form, and at this stage there is usually invasion of the dermis at one or more points and sometimes invasion of the epidermis. The proliferation of melanocytes in Hutchinson's melanotic freckle is most prominent around the skin appendages, particularly the hair follicles, and the invading nodules are usually composed of spindle cells of low-grade mitotic activity. More malignant cells are sometimes found but seldom is there grade 3 mitotic activity.

Hutchinson's melanotic freckle is more common in women than in men, and similarly, melanoma arising in Hutchinson's melanotic freckle is more common in women than in men. It is very unusual for melanoma arising in Hutchinson's melanotic freckle in a woman to give rise to metastases (McGovern, 1970). In men, however, metastases sometimes occur in tumours of grades 2 and 3 mitotic activity which have penetrated into the reticular dermis or beyond.

Melanoma with an adjacent intra-epidermal component of superficial spreading type (Figs. 1.2 and 1.3)

This type of melanoma commences as a flat macular lesion and sooner or later a recognisable nodule appears which represents invasion of the dermis. These tumours are usually black or dark brown in colour. The outline of these lesions is far better defined than the outline of Hutchinson's melanotic freckle. The margins of these lesions are usually palpable, whereas in Hutchinson's melanotic freckle the spreading margin is usually not palpable unless there are nodules of invasion. These lesions are usually smaller than Hutchinson's melanotic freckle and frequently are no more than between 1 and 2 cm in diameter, although on occasion they can be quite as extensive as a Hutchinson's melanotic freckle. They, too, may undergo spontaneous regression causing irregularities in the outline of the lesion (McGovern, 1975). Melanoma of this type can occur on any part of the body but is most

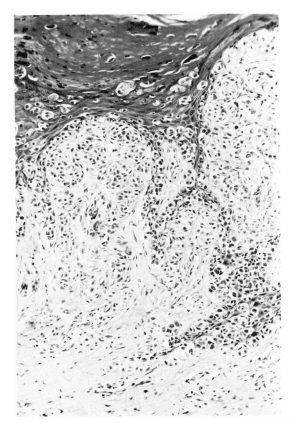

Fig. 1.2   Male aged 40 years with a melanoma arising in left ankle. There had been no antecedent blemish.

a. There is invasive melanoma in the dermis, and melanoma cells have invaded the overlying epidermis in a Pagetoid manner. H & E × 120.

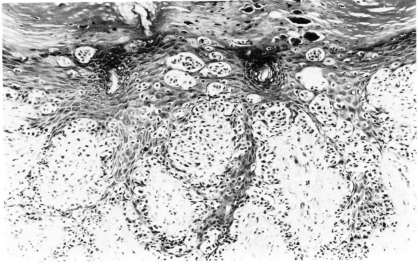

b. The spreading pigmented macule adjacent to the nodule is composed of proliferated basal melanocytes and clumps of melanoma cells invading the overlying epidermis. This is superficial spreading melanoma. H & E × 120.

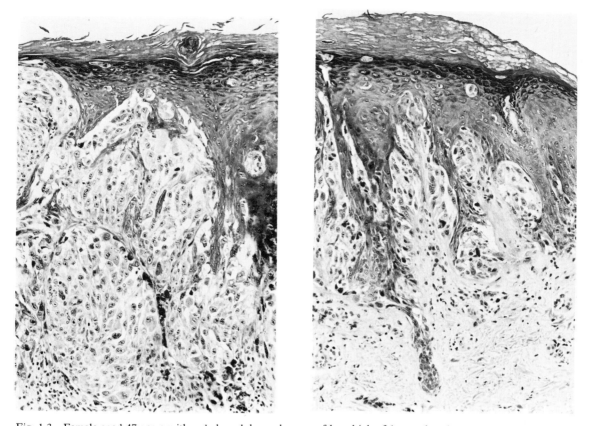

Fig. 1.3   Female aged 47 years with a dark nodular melanoma of her thigh of 1 year duration.
  a. Melanoma invading the dermis with very little invasion of the epidermis. H & E × 120.
  b. The adjacent superficial spreading melanoma consists of proliferated junctional cells with very little invasion of the epidermis. H & E × 120.

frequently found in the exposed parts. It is very unusual to find associated solar degeneration of the skin to the same extent as in Hutchinson's melanotic freckle.

The covered parts of the body may also be involved with melanoma of this type, and it can also involve various mucosae such as the conjunctiva, the mouth, the anal canal, the vulva and penis.

Microscopic appearances

Microscopically this lesion is characteristic. In addition to the invasion of the dermis by malignant melanocytes there is invasion of the epidermis (Figs. 1.2 and 1.3). The term 'superficial spreading melanoma' is used not to mean that there is spread within the epidermis but to mean that there is a wave of malignancy spreading out from a centre and transforming the melanocytes in the basal region, which thereupon invade both the epidermis and the dermis. This occurs in varying degrees so that in some cases the amount of intra-epidermal invasion may be slight and instead of this there is a continuous proliferation with cluster formation in the basal region of the epidermis. There may be in these cases some difficulty in distinguishing the lesion from Hutchinson's melanotic freckle, but this difficulty is not very commonly encountered because it is very unusual for there to be severe solar degeneration of the dermis or solar atrophy of the epidermis and its appendages in association with this type of melanoma.

Occasionally specimens are submitted to the pathologist in which superficial spreading melanoma is present without invasion of the dermis. This is very uncommon and if enough sections are taken micro-invasion, at least, is usually found.

Melanoma without an adjacent intra-epidermal component (Fig. 1.4)

This type of melanoma appears as a nodule and is sometimes called nodular melanoma (Clark, 1967). It has no surrounding pig-

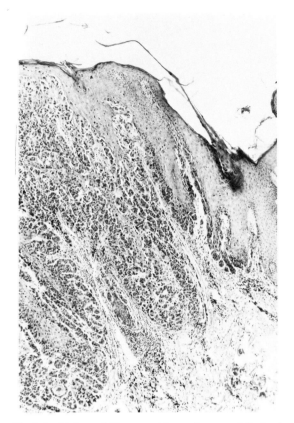

Fig. 1.4   Male aged 52 years with a melanoma of the back of 1 year duration. There is proliferation of melanocytes in the basal region of three of the rete ridges adjacent to the main mass of tumour. This is within the limits for including this tumour in the category 'without an adjacent intra-epidermal component'. H & E × 48.

mented macule. It may be polypoid and ulcerated and it is usually faster growing than melanomas of other types. It occurs in both exposed and unexposed skin and also in various mucosae such as the conjunctiva, the mouth, oesophagus, anal canal, vulva, vagina and penis.

Microscopic appearances

This tumour has minimal involvement in the adjacent epidermis (Fig. 1.4). The International Committee of Pathologists (McGovern *et al.*, 1973) recommended that melanomas with involvement of no more than three rete ridges should be included in this category. With involvement of more than three ridges, the tumour should be categorised as having an adjacent intra-epidermal component of superficial spreading type.

Tumours in this category are much more active than tumours of the other histogenetic types. They are more frequently of grades 2 or 3 mitotic activity and at the time of surgery have usually penetrated deeper (McGovern, 1970; McGovern, 1972). Most pedunculated or polypoid tumours are of this type and though there may be a large bulk of very active melanoma they cannot be satisfactorily staged because they pull the papillary zone of the dermis up above the level of the dermis. Little (1972) found approximately 60 per cent of patients with polypoid lesions had died within five years.

Relationship of 'moles' to melanoma

Whether or not there has been a pre-existent naevus, melanoma apart from that arising in a blue naevus arises in one of the three histogenetic patterns outlined above. When a melanoma commences in a junction naevus it is usually a melanoma with a component of superficial spreading type, and in the transformation of this naevus into melanoma the typical histological appearance of a naevus is lost, so that in most cases it is not possible on histological grounds to state whether or not there had been a junction naevus present. In many cases, however, there is evidence of a pre-existent naevus in that there are intradermal naevus cells associated with the melanoma. This leads to the supposition that there had been a compound naevus present from which the melanoma had developed.

Validity of the classification of melanoma

Clark *et al.* (1969) showed in the Northern Hemisphere that melanoma arising in Hutchinson's melanotic freckle has the best prognosis. Melanoma with no intra-epidermal component has the worst prognosis and melanoma with an adjacent intra-epidermal component of superficial spreading type occupies an intermediate position.

Survival rates in Australia (McGovern, 1970) are similar to those in the United States, as can be seen in Table 1.1. in which the figures for Boston are compared with those for Sydney.

Mitotic activity

It has been shown that survival rate can be correlated with the degree of mitotic activity (McGovern, 1972). We have used the system which was later recommended by the International Group of Pathologists (McGovern *et al.*, 1973). Their recommendation was that there should be three grades of mitotic activity:

1. Fewer than one mitosis per five high power fields;
2. Between one per five high power fields and one in each high power field;
3. One per high power field and over.

The figures are obtained using a 300 times magnification.

Levels of invasion

The levels of invasion were divided into five groups.

1. Intra-epidermal.
2. Papillary-dermal.
3. Papillary-reticular dermal interface.
4. Reticular-dermal.
5. Subcutaneous fat.

It has been observed, both in the Boston series and in the Sydney series, that the levels of invasion can be correlated with prognosis (Clark *et al.*, 1969; McGovern, 1970). Metastases were never observed arising from a tumour which was purely intra-epidermal. The survival rates in the present series are shown in Table 1.1.

One of the difficulties in the histological staging of melanoma according to the anatomical level is that the papillary zone varies in thickness. A melanoma may fill the papillary

Table 1.1   Five-year percentage survival according to histogenetic pattern

	Boston (Clark, 1967)	Sydney (McGovern, 1970)
1[a]	89·7	80
2[b]	68·5	70
3[c]	43·9	53

[a] Melanoma associated with Hutchinson's melanotic freckle.
[b] Melanoma with superficial spreading component.
[c] Melanoma with no intra-epidermal component.

layer depressing the reticular zone downwards instead of invading it. In this way a tumour at level 3, the papillary-reticular dermal interface, may be twice the depth of a tumour which has penetrated to level 4, the reticular zone. This anomaly has been resolved by Breslow (1970), who using an ocular micrometer found that he could correlate the survival rate with thickness of the tumour. This has been confirmed by Hansen and McCarten (1974) who found, in addition, that routine lymph node resection improved the survival rate of tumours measuring more than 1·5 mm in greatest depth, from 50 per cent with 5-year survival to 80 per cent, whereas routine lymph node resection had no significant effect upon survival in tumours less than 1·5 mm in greatest depth. In a subsequent study, Breslow (1975) found that tumours up to 0·75 mm in thickness, measuring from the granular layer of the epidermis to the deepest plane of invasion, had a good prognosis, and even if they penetrated to level 3 their prognosis was similar to that of lesions confined to level 2. Tumours measuring 0·76 mm up to 1·50 mm had an unpredictable prognosis with 70 per cent survival rate whether or not the lymph nodes were resected. Tumours more than 1·50 mm in depth had only 31 per cent survival rate, but lymph node resection increased the survival rate to 64 per cent.

While these figures are very convincing, other factors must also be taken into account when assessing prognosis. Amongst these is the sex of the patient, since women have a much better survival rate than men. The histogenetic pattern is important also, because melanomas in Hutchinson's melanotic freckle have a much better prognosis than other types of melanoma, and such tumours have been seen in women which have penetrated the subcutaneous fat yet have not metastasised. Furthermore, the difference in prognosis between tumours of different mitotic activity should be correlated with the depth of invasion.

Vascular invasion

Vascular invasion whether of blood or of lymphatic vessels is difficult to recognise owing to shrinkage of tissue, though we know that lymphatic vessel invasion must be a very frequent occurrence.

SPONTANEOUS REGRESSION OF NAEVI AND MELANOMAS

Regression in naevi

It is well known that naevi may disappear spontaneously and that, especially in children, the regressing naevus may be surrounded by a depigmented halo. The halo naevus was originally described by Sutton (1916) as leukoderma acquisitum centrifugum, an unusual form of vitiligo, but it was not until 1957 that Findlay published its histological features. Frank and Cohen (1964) amplified this and described 34 examples of halo naevi in 16 patients.

Microscopic appearances

Most halo naevi are compound naevi. During the active phase there is a dense lymphocytic infiltrate amongst the dermal naevus cells which become difficult to recognise and disappear. The junctional clusters take longer to disintegrate. When the naevus has disappeared, the lymphocytes disappear and fibrosis ensues. The resulting scar may be pale or dark depending on the amount of pigment in the original lesion. The affected melanocytes in the surrounding depigmented skin, the halo, are found with electron-microscopy to have lost their melanogenic organelles.

Regression in melanoma (Figs. 1.5, 1.6, and 1.7)

Melanoma, too, undergoes spontaneous regression and this is thought to account for the occurrence of metastatic melanoma in the absence of a demonstrable primary growth. The category 'primary site unknown' which is found in every large series of melanoma varies from 4·6 per cent of cases in the Queensland Melanoma Project (Beardmore, 1972) to 8·3 per cent in a series from Texas (Smith and Stehlin, 1965). The cause of this type of presentation was the source of much speculation until Smith and Stehlin described nine cases in which there was good histological evidence for spontaneous regression of the primary growth to have taken place. Since then it has been established that partial regression is not an uncommon phenomenon and is present in about 13 per cent of all melanomas (Little, 1972; McGovern, 1975). Nobody knows how many tumours undergo complete regression since very few sites of those which have regressed completely without giving rise to metastases are surgically removed.

Histological appearances

The phenomenon of spontaneous regression in melanoma is identical with the phenomenon of regression in naevi (McGovern, 1975). It is characterised by a dense infiltrate of lymphocytes which forms a continuous band beneath the portion of the tumour which is undergoing regression. These lymphocytes penetrate much further into the tumour than is seen in melanomas which are not undergoing regression. The tumour cells become indistinct and gradually disappear (Figs. 1.5 and 1.6). The process may halt at any time before the tumour has been completely destroyed, whereupon the lymphocytes disappear and are replaced by fibrosis in which there are prominent small blood vessels. Pigment-containing phagocytes are present in variable numbers according to the degree of pigmentation in the original lesion. Frequently there are foci of surviving melanoma cells and these can give rise to nodules of tumour subsequently. Surviving melanoma cells in the basal layer of the epidermis may also undergo proliferation after the process of regression has subsided and may

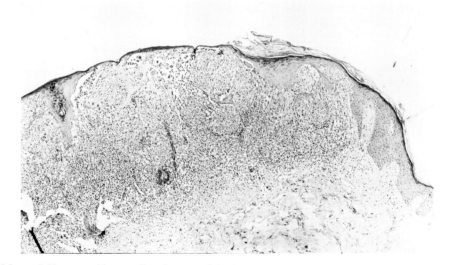

Fig. 1.5 Male aged 29 years with a small melanoma of thigh.
  a. There is a melanoma present which is very indistinct because it merges with a dense infiltrate of lymphocytes. H & E × 48.

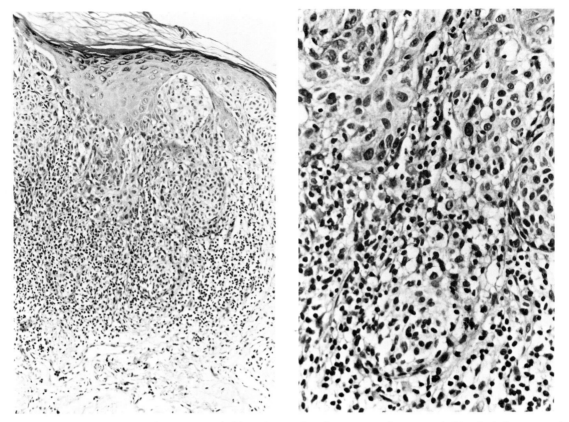

Fig. 1.5 b. A higher power shows a recognisable melanoma but the tumour cells surrounded by the inflammatory infiltrate are becoming indistinct. H & E × 120.

c. High power photomicrograph shows degenerating tumour cells amidst the lymphocytes. H & E × 300.

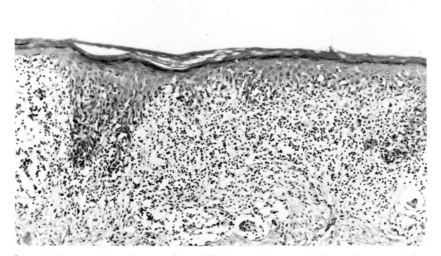

Fig. 1.6 Female aged 42 years with melanoma of arm. This is a melanoma which has almost entirely regressed except for the tumour cells in the epidermis, which are very degenerate. Note the dense lymphocytic infiltrate. H & E × 120.

continue to grow without the restraining influence of the phenomenon of regression from which they have just survived.

Type of melanoma involved in regression

Regression is common in Hutchinson's melanotic freckle and can also occur in the nodules of invasive melanoma which arise in the freckle. It is common also in the intra-epidermal component of superficial spreading type and less common in the nodule of melanoma accompanying the superficial spreading melanoma. Approximately one-third of all melanomas accompanied by an adjacent intra-epidermal component of superficial spreading type exhibit partial regression. Regression is very uncommon in melanomas without any adjacent intra-epidermal component.

Clinical appearances

Partial regression of melanoma results in a variety of clinical appearances depending upon the form of the melanoma, the extent of regression, and the degree of tumour destruction. The presence of regression does not mean that the prognosis has been altered; metastases may have already been established.

There are seven main clinical manifestations resulting from the regression process (McGovern, 1975; McGovern, 1976):

1. INFLAMMATORY NODULE WITH OR WITHOUT PIGMENTATION

Patients who have this manifestation of regression in a melanoma usually present because of enlarged lymph nodes which are found on histological examination to contain malignant melanoma. A search in the area drained by these lymph nodes may then reveal an inflammatory nodule. Such a nodule should be removed so that no surviving melanoma cells may remain.

2. PARTIAL REGRESSION OF MELANOMA WITHOUT SCARRING

Scarring is minimal or even imperceptible when regression occurs in superficial spreading melanoma confined to the epidermis (in-situ) or melanoma with early invasion of the dermis. In such cases the irregular shape and the pallor of the affected area indicate that regression has taken place or is in process.

Regression in melanomas with a very large intra-epidermal component of superficial spreading type may result in the irregular outlines similar to those of melanoma with an intra-epidermal component of Hutchinson's melanotic freckle type. However, the margins of superficial spreading melanoma are usually palpable whereas the margins of a Hutchinson's melanotic freckle are usually impalpable.

3. PARTIAL REGRESSION OF MELANOMA WITH SCARRING

Scarring occurs when melanoma which has invaded the dermis undergoes regression. If the regression is partial, the melanoma will be altered in shape by a pale scar or by several scarred areas. In some cases the entire superficial spreading component of a melanoma is obliterated so that the nodule which remains simulates melanoma with no intra-epidermal component.

4. PIGMENTED FOCUS WITH DEPIGMENTED HALO

This type of pattern may result in a lesion that simulates the halo naevus. However, it is usually larger, and in many cases there is peripheral pigmentation due to the regressing process having ceased before reaching the outer limits of the intra-epidermal component.

5. MELANOMA DIVIDED INTO SEVERAL ISLANDS

Sometimes the regression process affects different areas in a melanoma with a large intra-epidermal component of superficial spreading type, resulting in an appearance of multicentricity.

6. PIGMENTED SCAR

Whenever the pathologist receives a skin biopsy with a pigmented scar, his thoughts should instantly turn to the possibility of regressed melanoma. The entire specimen should be blocked and each block cut at different levels. In this way surviving melanoma cells may be found, which will confirm the diagnosis.

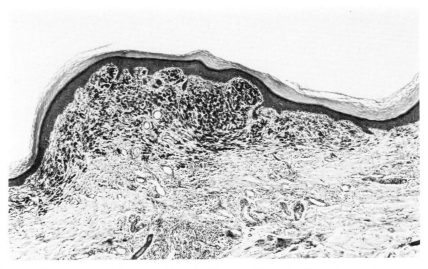

Fig. 1.7   A pigmented lesion removed from the thigh of a 25-year-old female. There is vascular scar tissue and a fairly dense collection of pigment-containing phagocytes. H & E × 48.
    This was diagnosed as the site of a regressed melanoma. The patient subsequently developed metastases.

7. METASTATIC MELANOMA WITH NO DEMON- STRABLE PRIMARY GROWTH

This type of presentation of melanoma has been found in approximately 7 per cent of cases. The site of the primary growth should be looked for, and if found it should be removed because it is quite possible that it may contain surviving melanoma cells capable of growth and metastases.

Prognosis in regressing melanomas

Mitotic activity and depth of invasion are the two most important parameters in the determination of prognosis in melanoma.

Mitotic activity in regressing melanoma is depressed and consequently the absence of mitoses does not mean that one is dealing with a low-grade tumour. It is quite possible for such a tumour to have given rise to metastases before regression had commenced and the metastases to be of grade 3 mitotic activity.

In assessing the depth of invasion in regressing melanoma one must assume that invasion had occurred to the deepest level of the inflammatory infiltrate. Since the deep level of the inflammatory reaction in regressing

melanoma is usually very well demarcated, this should present no difficulty.

Whereas metastases from a melanoma confined to the papillary layer of the dermis are unlikely, a similar tumour with a dense inflammatory infiltrate extending to a deeper level is in all probability a regressing melanoma that may have already metastasised.

The nature of regression

The regressive process in melanoma is confined to the skin. Metastases in the internal viscera do not seem to undergo regression, but metastases in skin may do so. The process is concerned with lymphocytes, probably T-lymphocytes, and its cessation before the tumour has been completely destroyed could be explained by the development of a state of anergy. The anergic state in which patients lose certain immune responses, particularly those related to delayed sensitivity reactions, may occur in patients with cancer of various types. Thornes *et al.* (1974) found by chance that induced proteolysis in an anergic patient with lung cancer enhanced skin tests for delayed hypersensitivity. In a subsequent study

(Thornes, 1974) it was found that although the effect was temporary, the use of streptokinase or a protease derived from *Aspergillus oryzae* converted anergic cancer patients to the reactive allergic state and that when the conversion was prolonged, clinical improvement occurred, but with reversion to the anergic state measureable advancement in growth of the tumour ensued.

It seems likely that the phenomenon of spontaneous regression in melanoma represents an enhancement of the immune mechanism and its cessation signifies reversion to the anergic state. Why the process is confined to the skin is inexplicable.

FROZEN SECTION IN THE DIAGNOSIS OF MALIGNANT MELANOMA

Many pathologists and some clinicians are apprehensive concerning the accuracy of frozen section examination for the diagnosis of malignant melanoma. However, our experience and that of other workers in Australia (Milton and Jelihovsky, 1962; McGovern, 1967; Hirst, McCarthy and Bale, 1972; Little and Davis, 1974; McGovern, 1976) has shown that frozen section is a very reliable method of diagnosis. We believe that it is very important to establish the diagnosis histologically before embarking upon any radical or disfiguring surgery, and that frozen section is the most expeditious way of doing this.

Frozen section diagnosis enables the surgeon to plan the complete operation. In the case of melanoma he can re-excise the site of the lesion and if necessary graft it in one operation. Not only does frozen section supply the diagnosis of melanoma, but also the histogenetic type, its mitotic activity and depth of invasion (Fig. 1.8). With this information he can decide whether or not to remove clinically uninvolved lymph nodes.

The frozen section specimen should consist of the whole lesion where feasible, with a narrow rim of normal skin. Should the lesion be very extensive and there be a possibility that total excision will not be the definitive treatment, a biopsy may be performed, taking care to select a nodule or that part of the lesion which seems likely to have invading tumour.

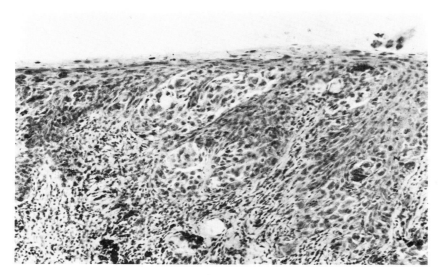

Fig. 1.8   Frozen section of an invasive melanoma with an adjacent intra-epidermal component of superficial spreading type.

a. The edge of the lesion showing superficial spreading melanoma. H & E × 120.

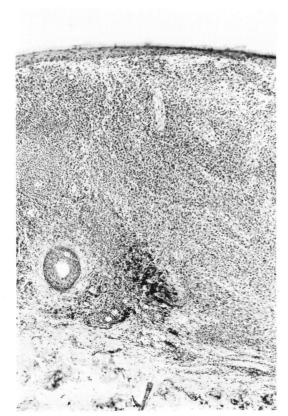

Fig. 1.8 b. The main mass of invading melanoma extending into the reticular zone of the dermis. The tumour measured 4 mm in depth in this part. H & E × 48.

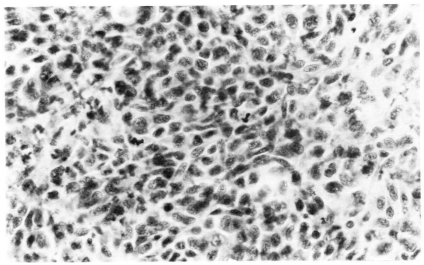

c. High power of the main mass of tumour showing type of cell and frequent mitoses. H & E × 300.

Comment: In this case frozen section revealed the histogenetic type of tumour, its level of invasion, and its mitotic activity.

It is desirable that the cryostat be used for frozen sections because, with care, it can give sections almost as good as paraffin sections. The sections should be mounted as permanent preparations. Even poor preparations should be kept permanently since subsequent paraffin sections of the frozen section block sometimes fail to show the invasive tumour seen in the frozen section.

Occasionally a definite diagnosis cannot be given and it is then necessary to await the paraffin sections. Deferred diagnoses of this type occur in about 4 to 6 per cent of cases (Little and Davis, 1974). False negative diag-noses are likely to be made by the inexperi-enced because of the difficulty in frozen sec-tions of distinguishing malignant melanocytes in the epidermis from keratinocytes in early lesions. False positive diagnoses, however, should be an extreme rarity.

There are several conditions which resemble malignant melanoma clinically. The com-monest of these are seborrhoeic keratoses, pig-mented basal cell carcinomas and thrombosed angiomas. These all have distinctive histologi-cal pictures which are unlikely to be mistaken for melanoma (see Plates I–VII, facing p. 32).

REFERENCES

Allen, A. C. & Spitz, S. (1953) Malignant melanoma: a clinicopathological analysis of the criteria for diagnosis and prog-nosis. *Cancer*, **6**, 1.

Anderson, D. E., Smith, J. L. & McBride, C. M. (1967) Hereditary aspects of malignant melanoma. *Journal of the American Medical Association*, **200**, 741.

Beardmore, G. C. (1972) The epidemiology of malignant melanoma in Australia. In *Melanoma and Skin Cancer. Proceedings of the International Cancer Conference, Sydney, 1972*, ed. McCarthy, W. H., p. 39. Sydney: Government Printer.

Black, H. S. & Lo, Wang-Bang (1971) Formation of a carcinogen in human skin irradiated with ultraviolet light. *Nature*, **234**, 306.

Bodenham, D. C. (1968) A study of 650 observed malignant melanomas in the south-west region. *Annals of the Royal College of Surgeons of England*, **43**, 218.

Boyd, W. (1966) *The Spontaneous Regression of Cancer*, Springfield, Ill.: Thomas.

Breslow, A. (1970) Thickness, cross-sectional areas and depth of invasion in the prognosis of cutaneous melanoma. *Annals of Surgery*, **172**, 902.

Breslow, A. (1975) Tumour thickness, level of invasion and lymph node dissection in stage 1 cutaneous melanoma. *Annals of Surgery*, **182**, 572.

Cawley, E. P. (1952) Genetic aspects of malignant melanoma. *Archives of Dermatology and Syphilology*, **65**, 440.

Central Cancer Registry, Melbourne, Victoria (1962) Report No. 2, *Cutaneous Melanoma*. Melbourne: Anti-Cancer Council of Victoria.

Clark, R. L. & MacDonald, E. J. (1953) The natural history of melanoma in man. In *Pigment Cell Growth*, p. 139. New York: Academic Press.

Clark, W. H., Jr (1967) A classification of malignant melanoma in man correlated with histogenesis and biologic behaviour. In *Advances in Biology of Skin*, ed. Montagna, W. & Hu Funan. Vol. 8, p. 621.

Clark, W. H., From, L., Bernadino, E. A., *et al.* (1969) The histogenesis and biologic behaviour of primary human melanomas of the skin. *Cancer Research*, **29**, 705.

Committee of Australian Pathologists (1967) Moles and malignant melanoma; terminology and classification. *Medical Journal of Australia*, **1**, 123.

Dubreuilh, M. W. (1912) De la mélanose circonscrite précancéreuse. *Annales de Dermatologie et Syphiligraphie*, **3**, 129.

Elwood, J. M. & Lee, J. A. H. (1974) Trends in mortality from primary tumours of skin in Canada. *Canadian Medical Association Journal*, **110**, 913.

Elwood, J. M., Lee, J. A. H., Walter, S. D., *et al.* (1974) Relationship of melanoma and other skin cancer mortality to latitude and ultraviolet radiation in the United States and Canada. *International Journal of Epidemiology*, **3**, 325.

Findlay, G. H. (1957) The histology of Sutton's naevus. *British Journal of Dermatology*, **69**, 389.

Fitzpatrick, T. B. & Breathnach, A. S. (1963) Das epidermale Melanin-Einheit-System. *Dermatologische Wochenschrift*, **147**, 481.

Frank, S. B. & Cohen, H. J. (1964) The halo nevus. *Archives of Dermatology*, **89**, 367.

George, P. A., Fortner, J. G. & Pack, G. T. (1960) Melanoma with pregnancy: a report of 115 cases. *Cancer*, **13**, 854.

Gordon, D., Silverstone, H. & Smithhurst, B. A. (1972) The epidemiology of skin cancer in Australia. In *Melanoma and Skin Cancer. Proceedings of the International Cancer Conference, Sydney, 1972*, ed. McCarthy, W. H., p. 23. Sydney: Government Printer.

Greeley, P. W., Middleton, A. F. & Curtin, J. W. (1965) Incidence of malignancy in giant pigmented nevi. *Plastic and Reconstructive Surgery*, **36**, 26.

Hansen, M. & McCarten, A. (1974) Tumor thickness and lymphocytic infiltration in malignant melanoma of the head and neck. *American Journal of Surgery*, **128**, 557.

Hirst, E., McCarthy, S. W. & Bale, P. M. (1972) Frozen section diagnosis of cutaneous malignancy. In *Melanoma and Skin Cancer. Proceedings of the International Cancer Conference, Sydney, 1972*, ed. McCarthy, W. H., p. 185. Sydney: Government Printer.

Hutchinson, J. (1892) Senile freckles. *Archives of Surgery*, **3**, 319.

Hutchinson, J. (1894) Lentigo-melanosis. A further report. *Archives of Surgery*, **5**, 252.

Kennedy, B. J. & Zelickson, A. S. (1963) Melanoma in an albino. *Journal of the American Medical Association*, **186**, 839.

Lancaster, H. O. (1956) Some geographical aspects of the mortality from melanoma in Europeans. *Medical Journal of Australia*, **1**, 1082.

Lancaster, H. O. & Nelson, J. (1957) Sunlight as a cause of melanoma. *Medical Journal of Australia*, **1**, 452.

Lane Brown, M. M. & Lelia, D. F. (1973) 'Celticity' and cutaneous malignant melanoma in Massachusetts. In *Pigment Cell. Mechanism in Pigmentation*, ed. McGovern, V. J. & Russell, P., p. 229. Basel: Karger.

Lane Brown, M. M., Thorpe, C. A. B., McMillan, D. S., et al. (1971) Genetic predisposition to melanoma and other skin cancers in Australians. *Medical Journal of Australia*, **1**, 852.

Lee, J. A. H. (1970) Fatal melanoma of the lower limbs and other sites: an epidemiologic study. *Journal of the National Cancer Institute*, **44**, 257.

Lee, J. A. H. (1972) Sunlight and the aetiology of malignant melanoma. In *Melanoma and Skin Cancer. Proceedings of the International Cancer Conference, Sydney, 1972*, ed. McCarthy, W. H., p. 83. Sydney: Government Printer.

Lee, J. A. H. (1973) The trend of mortality from primary malignant tumours of skin. *Journal of Investigative Dermatology*, **59**, 445.

Lee, J. A. H. & Carter, A. P. (1970) Secular trends in mortality from malignant melanoma. *Journal of the National Cancer Institute*, **45**, 91.

Lee, J. A. H. & Hill, G. B. (1970) Marriage and fatal malignant melanoma in females. *American Journal of Epidemiology*, **91**, 48.

Lee, J. A. H. & Issenberg, H. J. (1972) A comparison between England and Wales and Sweden in the incidence and mortality of malignant skin tumours. *British Journal of Cancer*, **26**, 59.

Lee, J. A. H. & Merrill, J. M. (1970) Sunlight and the aetiology of malignant melanoma: a synthesis. *Medical Journal of Australia*, **2**, 846.

Lewis, M. G. (1967) Malignant melanoma in Uganda. *British Journal of Cancer*, **21**, 483.

Little, J. H. (1972) Histology and prognosis in cutaneous malignant melanoma. In *Melanoma and Skin Cancer. Proceedings of the International Cancer Conference, Sydney, 1972*, ed. McCarthy, W. H., p. 107. Sydney: Government Printer.

Little, J. H. & Davis, N. C. (1974) Frozen section diagnosis of suspected malignant melanoma of the skin. *Cancer*, **34**, 1163.

MacDonald, E. J. (1959) Malignant melanoma among Negroes and Latin Americans in Texas. In *Pigment Cell Biology*, p. 171. New York: Academic Press.

MacDonald, E. J., Wolf, P. F. & Johnson, M. S. (1970) Regional patterns in morbidity from melanoma in Texas. *Journal of Investigative Dermatology*, **54**, 91.

McGovern, V. J. (1952) Melanoblastoma. *Medical Journal of Australia*, **1**, 139.

McGovern, V. J. (1966) Melanoblastoma in Australia. In *Structure and Control of the Melanocyte*, ed. Della Porta, G. & Mühlbock, O., p. 312. Berlin: Springer-Verlag.

McGovern, V. J. (1967) Malignant melanoma with particular reference to diagnosis by frozen section. *Bulletin of the Post-Graduate Committee in Medicine, University of Sydney*, **23**, 58.

McGovern, V. J. (1970) The classification of melanoma and its relationship with prognosis. *Pathology*, **2**, 85.

McGovern, V. J. (1972) Melanoma: growth patterns, multiplicity and regression. In *Melanoma and Skin Cancer. Proceedings of the International Cancer Conference, Sydney, 1972*, ed. McCarthy, W. H., p. 95. Sydney: Government Printer.

McGovern, V. J. (1975) Spontaneous regression in melanoma. *Pathology*, **7**, 91.

McGovern, V. J. (1976) *Malignant Melanoma. Clinical and Histological Diagnosis*. New York: John Wiley.

McGovern, V. J., Mihm, M. C., & 10 other authors (1973) The classification of malignant melanoma and its histologic reporting. *Cancer*, **32**, 1446.

McGuiness, B. W. (1963) Melanocyte-stimulating hormone: a clinical and laboratory study. *Annals of the New York Academy of Sciences*, **100**, 640.

Magnus, K. (1973) Incidence of malignant melanoma of the skin in Norway, 1955–1970. *Cancer*, **32**, 1275.

Mark, G. J., Mihm, M. C., Liteplo, M. G., et al. (1973) Congenital melanocytic nevi of the small and garment type. Clinical histologic and ultra-structural studies. *Human Pathology*, **4**, 395.

Milton, G. W. (1972) The diagnosis of malignant melanoma. In *Melanoma and Skin Cancer. Proceedings of the International Cancer Conference, Sydney, 1972*, ed. McCarthy, W. H., p. 95. Sydney: Government Printer.

Milton, G. W. & Jelihovsky, T. (1962) Frozen section examination in the diagnosis of cutaneous malignant melanoma (melanoblastoma). *Medical Journal of Australia*, **2**, 503.

Mori, W. (1973) Geographic pathology of malignant melanoma in Japan. In *Pigment Cell. Mechanisms in Pigmentation*, ed. McGovern, V. J. & Russell, P., p. 246. Basel: Karger.

Movshovitz, M. & Modan, B. (1973) Role of sun exposure in the etiology of malignant melanoma: epidemiologic inference. *Journal of the National Cancer Institute*, **51**, 777.

Norins, A. L. (1962) Free radical formation in the skin following exposure to ultra-violet light. *Journal of Investigative Dermatology*, **39**, 445.

Oettle, A. G. (1966) Epidemiology of melanomas in South Africa. In *Structure and Control of the Melanocyte*, ed. Della Porta, G. & Mühlbock, O., p. 292. Berlin: Springer-Verlag.

Pack, G. T., Davis, J. & Oppenheim, A. (1963) The relation of race and complexion to the incidence of moles and melanomas. *Annals of the New York Academy of Sciences*, **100**, 719.

Pack, G. T., Scharnagel, I. M. & Hillyer, R. A. (1952) Multiple primary melanoma. A report of 16 cases. *Cancer*, **5**, 1110.

Paget, J. (1864) Report of a clinical lecture on cases of tumours under moles. *Medical Times and Gazette*, **1**, 58.

Pathak, M. A. (1966) Photobiology of melanogenesis, biophysical aspects. In *Advances in Biology of Skin. The Pigmentary System*, ed. Montagna, W. & Hu, F. Vol. VIII, p. 397. London: Pergamon.

Peterson, N. C., Bodenham, D. C. & Lloyd, O. C. (1962) Malignant melanoma of the skin. A study of the origin, development, aetiology, spread, treatment and prognosis. *British Journal of Plastic Surgery*, **15**, 45.

Pringgoutoma, S. & Pringgoutoma, S. (1963) Skin Cancer in Indonesia. Biology of Cutaneous Cancer. *National Cancer Institute Monographs*, **10**, 191.

Reay-Young, P. S. & Wilkey, I. S. (1974) Tumours of the skin. In *The Epidemiology of Cancer in Papua New Guinea*, ed. Atkinson, L., Clezy, J. K., Reay-Young, P. S., *et al.*, p. 24. Papua New Guinea: Department of Public Health.

Reed, W. B., Becker, S. W., Jr, Becker, S. W., Sr, *et al.* (1965) Giant pigmented nevi, pigmented nevi, melanoma and leptomeningeal melanocytosis. *American Medical Association Archives of Dermatology*, **91**, 100.

The Registrar General's Statistical Review of England and Wales for the year 1965 (1970) *Supplement on Cancer*, p. 21. London: Her Majesty's Stationery Office.

Sampat, M. B. & Sirsat, M. V. (1966) Malignant melanoma of the skin and mucous membranes in Indians. *Indian Journal of Cancer*, **3**, 228.

Smith, J. L. & Stehlin, J. S. (1965) Spontaneous regression of primary melanoma with regional metastases. *Cancer*, **18**, 1399.

Sutton, R. L. (1916) An unusual variety of vitiligo (leukoderma acquisitum centrifugum). *Journal of Cutaneous Disease*, **34**, 797.

Thornes, R. D. (1974) Unblocking or activation of the cellular immune mechanism by induced proteolysis in patients with cancer. *Lancet*, ii, 382.

Thornes, R. D., Smith, H., Brown, O., *et al.* (1973) BCG plus protease I in malignant melanoma. *Lancet*, i, 1386.

Wallace, D. C. & Exton, L. A. (1972) Genetic predisposition to development of malignant melanoma. In *Melanoma and Skin Cancer. Proceedings of the International Cancer Conference, Sydney, 1972*, ed. McCarthy, W. H., p. 65. Sydney: Government Printer.

White, L. P., Linden, G., Breslow, L., *et al.* (1961) Studies on melanoma. *Journal of the American Medical Association*, **177**, 235.

2. Diagnosis, Differential Diagnosis and Biopsy

DIAGNOSIS

The following is a review of the clinical features of the patients in my (G. W. M.) series, suffering from either superficial spreading melanoma or nodular melanoma. Hutchinson's melanotic freckle is considered on page 29. The sex distribution was even with 50·9 per cent women and 49·1 per cent men. The age of the patients when they first observed the symptom leading to the diagnosis of melanoma varied between 5 and 85 years. Seventy-six per cent of patients were aged between 20 and 60 years, the average of all patients being 45·6 years. There was no difference between the age of men (45·8 years) and women (45·4 years) at the first symptom. Five and two-tenths per cent of the patients did not know whether the melanoma had developed from a pre-existing birthmark or skin blemish. However, in 29·3 per cent of the patients the melanoma developed *de novo* and was not preceded by any known 'mole', but two-thirds (65·5 per cent) knew of the existence of a skin blemish at the site at which the malignant melanoma developed. The duration of this pre-existing lesion was often hard to determine accurately because people do not always remember how long they have had their various 'moles'; but patients who observed a change in a pre-existing lesion noticed the premalignant condition for more than five years and often had been aware of the lesion since childhood. One patient developed malignancy in a large congenital dermal naevus, i.e. one known to be present at birth.

The first symptom noticed by the patient, as distinct from the symptom which made the patient go to his doctor, is shown as a percentage of each group in Table 2.1. The patient with a malignant melanoma usually observes the development or *change* of one or more of the four cardinal symptoms (Fig. 2.1):

1. *Growth.*
2. *Colour change.*
3. *Itch.*
4. *Bleeding.*

The commonest initial symptom was an increase in size, whether the melanoma developed *de novo* or in a pre-existing lesion. The lesion usually at first spreads out like an enlarging stain in the skin. This has been aptly called the horizontal growth phase by Clark *et al.* (1969). In other patients a brown mark originally flat became raised above the surrounding skin—the vertical growth phase.

The colour change usually appeared as a progressive darkening of the lesion. The

Table 2.1   The *first* symptom noticed by the patient (%). Shows in percentage the first symptoms observed by the patient which drew their attention to either the change in a pre-existing lesion or the development of a new lesion, which was ultimately diagnosed as a malignant melanoma. (For details see text)

	Men (%)	Women (%)	Mean (%)
Increase in size	45.0	50.1	47·5
Colour change	11·5	13·2	12·3
Itch	7·4	6·8	7·1
Bleeding	11·7	11·5	11·6
Pain	1·0	1·2	1·1
Lump	2·5	3·5	3·0
Scaling or crusting	1·0	1·4	1·2
Ulceration	1·8	1·6	1·7
No symptoms[a]	18·0	10·6	14·3

[a] 'No symptoms' implies that the lesion was first observed by someone else (doctor or relative), or that the primary lesion was not observed.

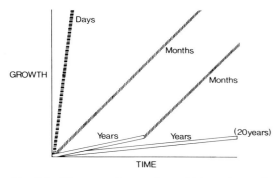

Fig. 2.1 Illustrates the speed at which a change in a melanoma may occur. In this case, the characteristic is defined as the size of the lesion, i.e. growth. The abscissa represents the different time scales for each line of the graph. The left-hand line marked 'days' illustrates a lesion which enlarges very rapidly (in a few days to approximately a week). Such lesions are usually infective and are unlikely to be malignant. The nearly horizontal line (20 years) illustrates the rate of change which may occur in a benign naevus. Characteristic rate of change in a malignant melanoma is illustrated by the lines labelled 'months', the left-hand side of which implies a lesion arising *de novo*, while the right-hand line illustrates a benign naevus that has become malignant.

darkening was often not uniform, and indeed in large junctional naevi the black discolouration almost always started in one part and then spread (Plate VIII*). The dark colour was often described as 'like a blood blister'. A loss of pigment may also be a feature of malignancy. The loss of colour occurs in one of two forms; in one, the growing tumour is either partly or wholly amelanotic; the other type of depigmentation is a variety of spontaneous regression (p. 16). If the regression is complete, a pale flat translucent scar may be all that remains at the site of the lesion (Plates X and XIII). Partial or complete regression of the primary lesion in this way does not imply that the disease is self-limiting, because there is still a considerable chance of metastasis developing in the draining lymph nodes or elsewhere.

The symptom of itch is characteristically mild, transient, and repetitive, i.e. it lasts for a few hours, disappears spontaneously and recurs from time to time. Patients often feel as if the irritation is not precisely in the pigmented area but rather in the surrounding skin and usually rub this area (i.e. the peripheral

* The plate section faces page 32.

skin) with the pulps of the fingers rather than scratch it.

Bleeding is another common symptom, and as a rule it is trivial in amount and the result of a trivial injury (Plate XI). The most frequent story is that the patient occasionally noticed a spot of blood on his clothing or a few flecks of blood on a towel when drying himself. The bleeding tended to be repeated with minor friction. This type of bleeding is different from that which occurs with a haemangioma which, if it bleeds at all, may drip blood for half an hour or more after an injury.

Pain is a rare symptom and is usually the result of a secondary infection or may be psychogenic. The symptom of lump referred to in Table 2.1 implies a palpable subcutaneous or lymph node metastasis. The scaling or crusting seen by patients takes one of two forms. As the malignant cells penetrate the epidermis, fine keratin flakes are displaced by the growing tumour (Plate VIII). At a later stage of the primary growth, bleeding or ulceration may lead to the formation of a coarse crust of congealed blood. Ulceration commonly occurs in large raised primary lesions where the surface has been abraded.

The presenting symptom which persuaded the patient to go to his doctor is shown in Table 2.2. The characteristics of the symptoms are the same as those given above. It can be seen that bleeding and itching, apart from increasing size, are the two most alarming symptoms.

If the lesion is situated on a site not often

Table 2.2 The presenting symptoms. Shows in percentages the symptoms which caused the patient to present to his doctor with a lesion which was ultimately diagnosed as a malignant melanoma. The remaining 13% consisted of patients who had an occult primary lesion and presented with symptoms of metastasis

	Men (%)	Women (%)	Mean (%)
Increase in size	37·2	40·9	39·1
Colour change	7·6	8·1	7·8
Itch	9·1	11·9	10·6
Bleeding	24·4	18·8	21·6
Pain	0·9	1·8	1·4
Lump	4·9	2·7	3·8
Scaling or crusting	2·1	2·1	2·1

inspected by the patient, e.g. the sole of the foot or the middle of the back, itching or bleeding are likely to draw the lesion to his attention.

Duration of symptoms

The duration of each of the symptoms from the time they were first noticed to the time the patient went to his doctor is shown in Table 2.2. This confirms the suggestion that bleeding and irritation cause the patient alarm, while increasing size and change of colour are often disregarded for a longer period. The number of patients who complain of pain, lump or scaling are small and the mean duration of the symptoms is therefore not as significant in the overall picture of the disease as might appear from these figures. More than three-quarters of the time interval between the first symptom and treatment resulted from the delay in presentation to the doctor (Table 2.3).

It has been suggested that trauma to a benign lesion may precipitate malignant degeneration. However, for reasons already mentioned on page 27, it appears more likely that trauma directs the patient's attention to an already malignant lesion rather than precipitate malignancy in an otherwise benign naevus. The history of trauma and of bleeding frequently went together. The hazard of partial biopsy is discussed on page 34.

It will be seen from all the figures given above that there is little if any difference in the symptomatology of primary malignant melanoma between men and women.

Special diagnostic problems

Three problems relating to the diagnosis of

Table 2.3   The mean duration of each of the main symptoms of the primary lesion in months

	Men (months)	Women (months)	Mean (months)
Increase in size	12·6	14·6	13·7
Colour change	11·4	11·5	11·5
Itch	7·5	6·8	7·1
Bleeding	4·5	7·2	5·9
Pain	4·8	3·7	4·1
Lump	8·3	9·2	8·7
Scaling or crusting	6·1	5·8	5·9

primary malignant melanoma remain to be considered: *multiple primary lesions, melanoma in pregnancy, and occult primary melanoma*. The diagnosis of these conditions will be considered here; other problems relating to them are dealt with in Chapter 11.

Multiple primary lesions are by no means rare (27 cases in this series with a total of 76 primary lesions) (McGovern, Milton and Maxwell, in press). The proof that multiple primary melanomas are each true primary lesions and not a single melanoma associated with metastases is established largely by histological criteria, i.e. the continuation of the primary growth with the basal layer of the epidermis, but supportive evidence is available from the clinical behaviour of the tumours. Widespread disease does not follow the appearance of a second primary melanoma which one would expect if the second lesion was a metastasis. The patient who develops multiple primary melanomas usually follows one of two patterns.

1. The lesions arise simultaneously but are widely separated, for example, one on the shoulder and another on the thigh (8 cases). The clinical history and their appearance is similar to single lesions.

2. A second primary melanoma may develop after the treatment of the first. The second or subsequent lesions are sometimes close to the site of the first, e.g. in the same limb (4 cases) or in distant parts of the body (15 cases). The symptoms of each lesion are in no way peculiar.

Two patterns of symptomatology of *primary melanoma in pregnancy* should be mentioned. Four women have been seen who described how a small non-pigmented or slightly brown lesion enlarged during pregnancy, and after delivery the lesion regressed leaving a small mark. The same enlargement of the lesion occurred with the next pregnancy, and in one patient this happened three times before the lesion was biopsied and found to be melanoma. One prominent symptom in the primary melanoma of pregnancy is itch, and for this reason any 'mole' which enlarges and develops an itch during pregnancy would be better excised.

Malignant melanoma with an occult primary lesion (Milton, Lane Brown and Gilder, 1967) accounted for 39 cases. The incidence of occult primary lesions is much higher in men (82 per cent) than in women (18 per cent). The reason for this disparity between sexes is not clear. The history of a patient with an occult primary melanoma follows one of several patterns.

1. The site of the lesion may be marked by a pale (amelanotic) scar or an area of slightly translucent skin. The patient may explain that this evolved by:

   a. A black skin lesion enlarged, became irritated and 'infected' (i.e. red and inflamed) and then completely disappeared.

   b. The lesion may have 'faded away' without any irritation for no apparent cause.

2. A 'blood blister' may have received some trivial injury which was followed by either a regression of the lesion or by it 'falling off'. In both instances the wound healed without trace of the original lesion. The longest interval recorded between a presumed primary lesion and the appearance of metastasis in this series was six years.

3. In other patients, no history suggestive of a primary lesion and no scar to mark its site was discovered.

4. Two patients were seen in whom a true occult primary lesion did not exist because each of them had what appeared to be an unaltered junctional naevus in the drainage area of metastatic lymph nodes. The lesion was excised and found to be malignant.

In these cases, if the primary lesion or its site was not discovered soon after the diagnosis was established by the demonstration of metastatic disease in lymph nodes, it was never found subsequently.

Clinical appearance

The clinical appearance of a malignant melanoma can vary greatly. In flat superficial spreading melanoma the lesion is usually dark brown or near black, the surface matt, the edge slightly irregular and the colour may be uniform or variable. The typical nodular melanoma is raised (3–5 mm), dark brown or black in the raised area. The surface is often glossy, but in small lesions the black, erupting mass of cells push the epidermis aside and so part of the periphery of the lesion may have fine keratin flakes of the displaced epidermis (Plate VIII). In larger lesions, the surface may be ulcerated or covered by small scabs of congealed blood. The average maximum diameter of the primary lesion in this series was approximately 2–3 cm. A malignant melanoma originating in a large junctional naevus may be partly surrounded by the remains of the pale brown benign precursor (Plate VIII). A halo around part of a melanoma may be one of four types:

1. A narrow (2 mm) inflammatory blush abutting the edge of the growing tumour which may represent a host reaction to the tumour. The halo tends to be more prominent if the lesion is irritating the patient.

2. A wide inflammatory halo results from ulceration and infection of the lesion (Plate VI).

3. A halo resulting from subepidermal spread of the melanoma cells was rare in this series and often takes the form of satellites with a clear margin of skin between the two.

4. A pale halo due to partial spontaneous regression has been referred to in the history, but as a rule this form of depigmentation is either patchy at the periphery or largely at the centre of the lesion (Plates II and V). A much rarer form of regression halo, seen only once in this series, is a complete circumferential halo of regression tumour (Plate IV).

Hutchinson's melanotic freckle (HMF)
(Plates VII and XIV)

Hutchinson's melanotic freckle (Hutchinson, 1892, 1894, 1896) is a disease entity different from either of the previously described forms of melanoma. The clinical history given by such a patient is that she will have noticed a flat, mottled freckle spreading slowly and haphazardly like a stain across the skin for as long as 10 to 20 years (Plate XIV). As the lesion is more common in women than in men and is frequently, but not invariably, on the face, the patient often learns to conceal the discolouration with cosmetics. Apart from the colour, the lesion will have caused no symptoms throughout this prolonged horizontal growth phase.

The duration of the horizontal growth phase is variable, but after about 10 years (Molesworth, 1965; McGovern and Lane Brown, 1969, D) a vertical growth phase usually begins and the lesion develops a lump which then grows in a matter of months. The freckle near the area may have a fine crusty surface while the lump may be darkly pigmented, although it is often amelanotic as in one of Hutchinson's original cases.

On examination, the appearance is characteristic. The serpentine edge usually sharply separates the coloured from the normal skin. The colour of the lesion itself varies considerably in different areas and the patient may describe how one part of the freckle darkened while another became pale. The hair follicles and skin surface texture are normal until the vertical growth phase commences and when this happens the nodule is soft as in other types of melanoma. In older people there may be obvious skin solar damage in the surrounding areas, but even in younger patients with HMF the microscope reveals solar atrophy of the epidermis and collagen degeneration in the dermis (McGovern and Lane Brown, 1969, D). This degree of solar degeneration is not common with melanomas of other types but is invariable with HMF. Distant metastasis rarely occur with HMF, even when the nodular or invasive stage is reached (McGovern and Lane Brown, 1969, E; Clark *et al.*, 1969; Molesworth, 1965).

DIFFERENTIAL DIAGNOSIS

The causes of localised discolouration of the skin may be divided into:

1. *Melanin*
2. *Blood*
   a. in venous spaces.
   b. in arterial spaces.
   c. extravascular.
3. *Applied colours*, e.g. cosmetics, tattooing, dirt.

Localised pigmentation due to melanin

FRECKLE (EPHELIS)

Freckles are probably the commonest of all skin pigmentations in pale-skinned races and are especially marked in people of reddish complexion who tan poorly. Freckles are not usually present at birth but increase during childhood. Freckles darken after solar exposure, at or near puberty and during pregnancy. They are flat and impalpable. Clinically and pathologically there is little distortion of the skin architecture and the lesion therefore appears to be almost as much a functional abnormality as a structural change.

JUNCTIONAL NAEVUS (Plates XV and XVI)

These are not usually present at birth but develop either in early infancy or childhood. Junctional naevi usually remain unchanged for long periods although the observant or anxious patient may notice a slight enlargement over the years, especially in children near puberty. This enlargement may cause anxiety but two features can be reassuring. Junctional naevi are often multiple and the parent may observe that all the 'brown marks' enlarge as the child grows. The rate of change is measured in years and not months. Clinically, a junctional naevus is a flat, brown stain in the skin, and even when examined with a hand lens the fine skin lines and pores are intact. Although usually pale brown, junctional naevi are occasionally quite dark but rarely black. A junctional naevus consists of a proliferation of melanocytes at the derm-epidermal junction, i.e. in the immediate vicinity of the basement membrane of the epidermis. The proliferation is not excessive and so the lesion is usually, if not always, impalpable.

COMPOUND NAEVUS (Plate XVII)

The history of a compound naevus is similar to that of a junctional naevus. The distinction between the two is made on clinical examination. The proliferation of melanocytes in a compound naevus is more extensive than in a junctional naevus, and so the superficial part of the dermis is expanded and the surface is raised.

DERMAL NAEVUS (Plates XVIII and XIX)

Dermal naevi often develop by the maturation of either junctional or compound naevi; it follows that the majority of naevi in old age are dermal naevi. The usual history, therefore, is one of very slow change, even in those dermal naevi which arise *de novo*. A dermal naevus consists, as one might expect, of a further development of the melanocytes which now lie in the dermis. Dermal naevi are common about the face, they are raised, easily palpable and frequently have abnormal hair follicles. Dermal naevi have been known for centuries. Don Quixote's skin blemish with 'bristles' sticking out of it was almost certainly a dermal naevus and the 'warts' in the death mask of Oliver Cromwell are dermal naevi. However, another less common form of dermal naevus is a true congenital deformity, i.e. it is present at birth and may be very large—the so-called 'bathing trunk' naevus (Plate XXI).

HALO NAEVUS (Plate XXII)

This is usually noticed in adolescence and because the halo is most obvious when the adjacent skin is tanned, the patient frequently visits his doctor in the early summer accompanied by an anxious parent. The halo naevus remains virtually unchanged for months, up to a few years, and then regresses leaving no residual scar. The central portion is usually pale brown but the striking feature of the lesion is a circular or elliptical area of total depigmentation having a precise border with the normal suntanning around it. The depigmented halo will be unaffected by solar exposure and will blister and burn without subsequent pigmentation. A halo naevus is virtually never malignant and does not require excision.

The non-pigmented halo is of interest because the melanocytes in this area are devoid of melanosomes but otherwise resemble normal melanocytes. The base beneath the central compound naevus area has marked lymphocytic infiltration, presumably an inflammatory reaction or host rejection (McGovern and Lane Brown, 1969, F; Jacobs *et al.*, 1975). The borders of the halo are always so well defined that it appears as if some melanogenic inhibitor diffuses from the central part of the lesion into the surrounding skin. On rare occasions (once in this series) a primary malignant melanoma may have a completely circular depigmented halo.

BLUE NAEVUS (Plate XXIII)

A blue naevus remains unchanged for years and can look alarming if the surface is wiped off by severe injury and the black glossy mass of the densely packed melanocytes in the dermis appear sinister. The clues to the correct diagnosis are the static history and the severity of the injury needed to abrade the surface. Blue naevi are often small (i.e. less than 0·5 cm diameter), raised a few millimetres and a blue-black colour. The uninjured surface appears to be normal epidermis stretched over a dark mass beneath.

Before leaving the subject of naevi, one further aspect of these lesions requires elaboration. The clinical features of junctional naevi in adolescents has been mentioned as a darkening and possibly slight enlargement. Pathologically junctional naevi in childhood and especially adolescence can appear to be confusing and a variety of terms have been used to describe them; juvenile melanoma and Spitz naevus (Spitz, 1948) are the two commonest. The term 'active junctional naevus' is another variant of a similar pathological picture. Clinically these lesions all resemble the ordinary 'common or garden' junctional naevus under the influence of approaching or actual puberty. Pathologically, the cells are often spindle or epitheloid shaped and mitotic figures may be seen. These lesions are not malignant and do not require ablative surgical treatment. If there is the slightest doubt about the pathological diagnosis, two steps are necessary.

1. Careful preparation of quality paraffin sections.

2. The sections should be reviewed independently by at least two and preferably three experienced pathologists before a diagnosis of malignant melanoma is either rejected or considered established.

Melanin pigmentation can appear in other skin lesions, for example, pigmented basal cell carcinoma (Plate XXV). The pigmentation is the result of the growing basal cells being injected with melanin from adjacent melanocytes. I have no personal experience of pigmented squamous cell carcinoma (SCC) and from all accounts it is a very rare tumour. The growth and behaviour patterns are said to resemble those typical of SCC.

A more common difficulty arises with very rapidly growing squamous cell carcinomas which may resemble an amelanotic melanoma or a sarcoma (Lever, 1961). The distinction depends on even traces of melanin pigmentation. From the clinical point of view the distinction may not be of overriding importance, because the treatment of these conditions will be similar in curable lesions and ineffective in incurable ones.

SEBORRHOEIC KERATOSIS (Plates XXVI and XXVII)

This is a lesion common in the second half of life. The skin is often greasy, and the lesions multiple. In the early stages of development, the lesion may appear to have a somewhat glossy surface while at later stages it looks like the end of a dirty paint brush. The pigmentation may not be homogeneous and the surface may be cracked. The patient will give a history of single or multiple lesions remaining stationary over long periods. He may have noticed 'pieces fall out of the lesion' when he rubs it with a towel. If he has been observant he will also have noticed that when this occurs the lesion does not bleed. A seborrhoeic keratosis consists of large blocks of densely packed keratinised squamous epithelium.

Localised pigmentation due to blood

HAEMANGIOMA (Plates XXVIII and XXIX)

This will not be a complete discussion of the clinical diagnosis of haemangioma: I will only consider those few varieties which may be confused with malignant melanoma.

A venous (cavernous) haemangioma, especially on the lip, may superficially resemble a melanoma. The patient tells the history that his 'blemish' has remained unchanged for many years. On examination, the surface of the lesion

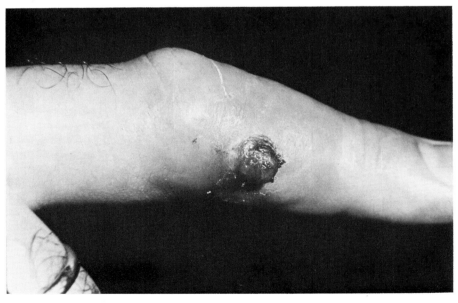

Fig. 2.2   A pyogenic granuloma. The rapidly developing, raised, red and inflamed looking lesion is commonly situated on the fingers but can grow at any site and is frequently surrounded by an inflammatory halo. Its most alarming feature—rapid growth measured in days—indicates that it is not a malignant melanoma.

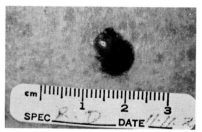

Plate I

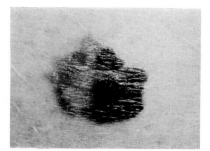

Plate II

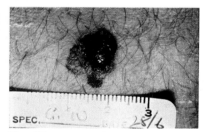

Plate III

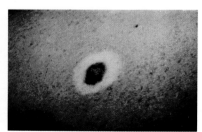

Plate IV

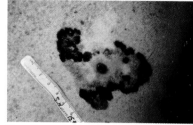

Plate V

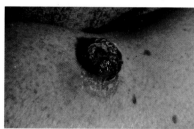

Plate VI

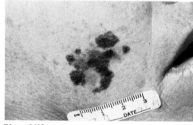

Plate VII

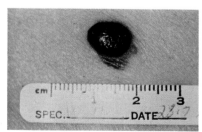

Plate VIII

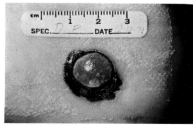

Plate IX

Plate I Superficial spreading melanoma varying in colour from brown to blue-black, with a reddish nodule of invasive melanoma arising in it.

Plate II Superficial spreading melanoma with an invasive nodule. Part of the superficial spreading component has undergone regression resulting in depigmentation.

Plate III A large dark nodule of melanoma with a small adjacent intra-epidermal component of superficial spreading type.

Plate IV A dark nodule of melanoma surrounded by depigmentation. This indicates regression. However, regression of the primary tumour did not influence the prognosis because this young man died in three years from disseminated melanoma.

Plate V A melanoma of superficial spreading type in which there are numerous small nodules of invasion. There has been partial regression leading to a very irregular outline and an appearance suggesting multicentricity.

Plate VI A polypoid melanoma with no adjacent intraepidermal component. Note the thick crusts of congealed blood on the surface of the lesion and the inflammatory halo near its upper part

Plate VII A typical Hutchinson's melanotic freckle with irregular outline due to partial regression and several nodules of invasive melanoma.

Plate VIII Illustrates a malignant melanoma, the upper portion of which is nodular and the lower portion is superficial spreading in type. Note the thin flakes of displaced epidermis on the surface of the nodular area which also has a glossy appearance. The superficial spreading area could be an area of junctional naevus from which the original lesion developed, as there is no destruction of the skin lines in this part. The history of the lesion would suggest this because a 'birth mark' had been present for many years and in the six months prior to the patient presenting with this lesion the upper pole of the 'birth mark' had started to grow rapidly.

Plate IX Malignant melanoma on the heel of a 12-year-old girl. Note: (1) Considerable central amelanotic growth on the upper surface of which the skin can be seen pushed away by the expansion. (2) The black epithelial invasion along the lower parts of the tumour.

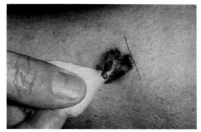

Plate X

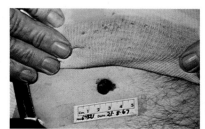

Plate XI

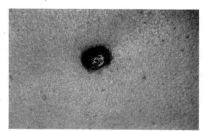

Plate XII

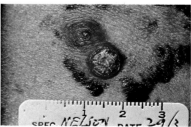

Plate XIII

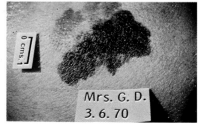

Plate XIV

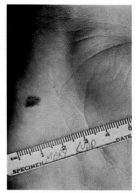

Plate XV

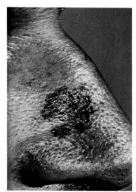

Plate XVI

Plate X Melanoma on the shin of an elderly woman. This lesion shows characteristics typical of melanoma. Clinical history had been one of growth measured over a period of months. The patient had also noticed that the lesion stuck to her stocking and when she took this off it bled a few drops of blood so she developed a habit of covering the lesion with cotton wool, as seen here. Part of the growth is nodular and it was in this area that the ulceration and bleeding occurred. The rest of it shows some areas of dark pigmentation and others of amelanotic growth while there are also areas of regression of part of the primary tumour.

Plate XI A raised nodular melanoma showing the type of bleeding commonly observed, i.e. trivial blood loss resulting from trivial trauma.

Plate XII This lesion is 1·5 cm in diameter (maximum) and raised about 3 mm. It is a nodular melanoma in which there is no superficial spreading component. Although the growth is almost entirely above the surface of the skin in a plateau formation the pores of the sweat glands are still detectable.

Plate XIII An unusual variety of malignant melanoma in which several patterns of growth and regression are demonstrable. This lesion is sometimes called a 'ring melanoma'. The peripheral black, expanding, growing edge is malignant and slightly raised above the surrounding skin. Behind this is an area of regression in which the central portion of the tumour has completely disappeared leaving normal skin architecture. However, two nodules of actively growing tumour are in the process of erupting through the skin near the centre of the lesion. This figure illustrates well that malignant melanoma is a multiple disease, the multiplicity being caused by cellular adaptation and evolution.

Plate XIV A typical Hutchinson's melanotic freckle. The following factors are characteristic: (1) It is on the cheek of a middle-aged to elderly woman. (2) Pigmentation is irregular and the edge is serpentine. (3) Nearly all the lesion is impalpable and the skin architecture appears normal. The clinical history of this patient indicated that the lesion had been present for 15 years and had slowly advanced in one area while regressing in another. If a nodule developed in this lesion, it could be either pigmented or amelanotic.

Plate XV Shows a freckle with possibly some areas of junctional naevus on the palm. The plate was chosen to illustrate the continuity of skin architecture characteristic of lesions with minimal structural change in the skin, i.e., freckles and junctional naevi.

Plate XVI A close-up photograph of a junctional naevus on the side of the nose. Note the intact pores and the flat impalpable lesion. The diagnostic feature of the history is that the lesion had remained static for many years.

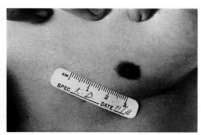

Plate XVII

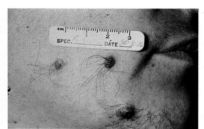

Plate XVIII

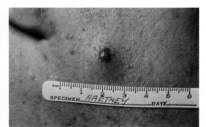

Plate XIX

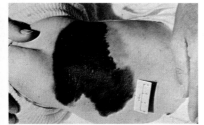

Plate XX

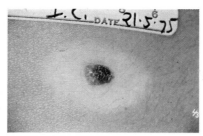

Plate XXII

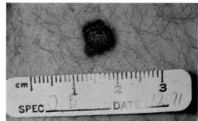

Plate XXIII

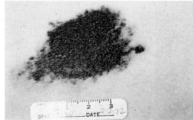

Plate XXIV

Plate XIX Dermal naevus on the face, associated with a sebaceous cyst. This lesion may cause alarm if the cyst becomes inflamed, whereupon it enlarges in a few days. However, the extreme rapidity of the enlargment is the most reassuring feature.

Plate XX A large congenital dermal naevus which enlarged as the patient grew. Extreme versions of this are known as 'bathing trunk' naevi (see Plate XXI).

Plate XXI Shows a 'bathing trunk' naevus of a baby. It is a true congenital deformity of the skin present at birth. It is difficult to estimate the risk of malignant change in such lesions but in the records of the Melanoma Clinic at Sydney Hospital, in 1800 patients suffering from malignant melanoma only one was known to have originated in such a lesion. However, the parent should be warned that if the lesion develops any lumps or nodules in it the patient should be immediately reassessed and when the child is old enough, provided the lesion is not too extensive, excision is the treatment of choice.

Plate XXII Shows a classical halo naevus. The central portion is a compound naevus and the periphery is marked by an amelanotic halo which always has a precise edge, almost as if the melanogenic inhibitor substance defused into the adjacent skin.

Plate XXIII A blue naevus. Note the intact epithelium appearing stretched over the accumulated pigment containing cells beneath. The lesion is usually, but not always, a blue-black colour. Any change in its texture or size is gradual.

Plate XXIV An unusual variant of the blue naevus known as the cellular blue naevus. It is present from early infancy, very dark in colour, the skin appears thickened and firmer than normal and the densely packed melanocytes can be seen extending beyond the edges of the obvious lesion. It is usually removed, not because of the risk of malignancy but because of its appearance.

Plate XVII A compound naevus on the breast. Note the distorted architecture in the central portion of the lesion which, nevertheless, is not ulcerated or flaked. The history, as with nearly all naevi, would have been one of negligible or very gradual change.

Plate XVIII Characteristic dermal naevi on the face; they are small and have been present since birth with very little change since then except for enlargement during early puberty. The patient is a young man of 17 years of age. Note the lesions are raised and there are long hairs protruding from their surface, and in at least two of them the pores of the skin are more prominent than normal. The characteristic feature to reassure the anxious parent of such a patient is that the change occurred in all three lesions simultaneously, at about the time of the onset of puberty. Such lesions may be removed for cosmetic purposes but the risk of malignancy in them is extremely small.

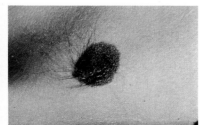

Plate XXI

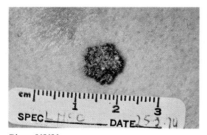

Plate XXV

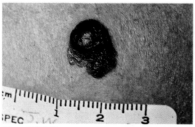

Plate XXVI

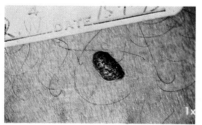

Plate XXVII

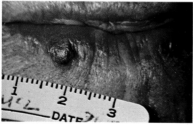

Plate XXVIII

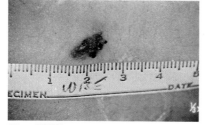

Plate XXIX

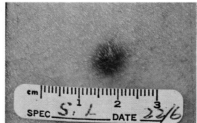

Plate XXX

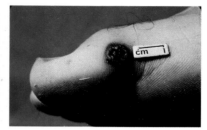

Plate XXXI

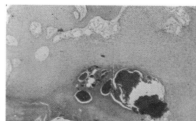

Plate XXXII

Plate XXV A pigmented basal cell carcinoma. The history helps to establish the diagnosis of this lesion; however, it will often have a pearly edge.

Plate XXVI A darkly pigmented seborrhoeic keratosis. Clinical appearance could be confused with malignant melanoma, but the clinical history is of a lesion unchanged for long periods. Note the waxy surface with pronounced pores. These lesions are commonly flatter with a more definite, greasy look.

Plate XXVII Seborrhoeic keratosis appearing almost like a greasy plaque stuck on the skin. A plane of cleavage can sometimes be developed which will split the mass off from the underlying tissue. These lesions occur in middle age and beyond and are commonly multiple.

Plate XXVIII A venous haemangioma on the lip. It is characteristically a bluish-purple colour and is stationary for many years. In this case, the lesion had been known to be unchanged for over 20 years. Note the intact surface.

Plate XXIX Shows a lobulated haemangioma on the arm. A haemangioma may closely resemble a malignant melanoma and no definitive treatment should be undertaken until the tissue diagnosis is established. The lesion shown above illustrates an important characteristic which will help to suggest the diagnosis, i.e. that the surface appears to be lobulated, although in most instances the lobules are smaller than those shown here.

Plate XXX Shows a characteristic sclerosing haemangioma which usually has a coppery colour. It is firmer than normal skin and firmer than a melanoma and the lesion often feels warm and firm to the touch. A melanoma always feels soft.

Plate XXXI Intraepithelial haemorrhage. This should cause no difficulty in diagnosis and a history of injury is usually obtained. The characteristic features are well-defined dark discolouration in the epidermis and if the epidermis is thick, as on the palms and sole, the skin lines are intact and cross the surface of the pigmented area. History of injury is usually obtainable with lesions on the hand, but on the foot a new pair of shoes may be enough to produce the haemorrhage.

Plate XXXII Histological appearance of the skin obtained from the patient in Plate XXXI. Note the haemorrhage into the thickened cornified epithelium of the foot. The gross architecture of such a lesion permits the diagnosis to be established with certainty on frozen section examination.

is intact and there is no evidence of mucosal invasion. Haemangiomas of this type are soft and compressible.

A more confusing form of venous haemangioma is in the skin rather than the mucosa and has large vascular spaces. It is either purple or black and although it may remain static for many years, it can closely resemble the appearance of a melanoma. The distinction between the two lesions is made on the following characteristics:

1. The static history.
2. If injured, the lesion will tend to bleed for prolonged periods (say 45 minutes) because of the large venous spaces.
3. In spite of the size of the lesion, the surface is intact and does not have the appearance of infiltration.
4. Although the lesion may be compressible, it may be surprisingly difficult to empty, but if this can be shown, the diagnosis is certain.

SCLEROSING HAEMANGIOMA (Plate XXX)

This is also known as hystocytoma and should not cause difficulty with melanoma but has been known to do so. They are static or slow-growing. In the early stages of development they often feel warm relative to the surrounding tissue, they feel firm because of their fibrous tissue content, and they do not bleed easily. Sclerosing haemangiomas have a coppery colour somewhat reminiscent of the early stages of a developing varicose eczema. They are not malignant and it is unnecessary to remove them, except possibly to allay anxiety.

PYOGENIC GRANULOMA (Fig. 2.2)

These are not true tumours but are a form of infected haemangioma. They are commonly situated about the fingers, but may occur anywhere. They cause considerable alarm because of the rapid growth rate; indeed this is the very thing which should indicate that they are benign because they will enlarge in the course of a few days to a week or so, which is too rapid for malignant melanoma. They are flesh coloured and often have a surrounding inflammatory halo larger than that associated with melanoma. Diagnosis is easily established

by excision biopsy which also constitutes adequate treatment.

INTRA-EPITHELIAL HAEMORRHAGE (Plates XXXI and XXXII)

This is unlikely to cause difficulty in the diagnosis of malignant melanoma except where it occurs on the palm or the sole. The lesion consists of bleeding in between the layers of the epithelium and consequently is usually noticed quite suddenly and the patient is often unaware of previous injury. Occasionally, they may have had a new pair of shoes which gives a clue to the diagnosis. The diagnosis can be made by the slight purple discolouration of the lesion and by biopsy.

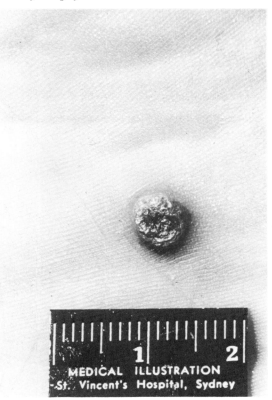

Fig. 2.3 The sole of the foot of an 8-year-old child who developed this rapidly growing ulcerated lesion over a course of eight days. The lesion followed the removal of a wooden splinter and the person who removed it had infective warts on the fingers—hence the lesion. The history of an eight-day growth is too rapid for malignant melanoma.

BIOPSY

A diagnostic test such as excision biopsy is valuable if it provides more precise information at an earlier stage of the disease than that obtained from clinical examination.

The reason for a skin biopsy or localised excision is usually one or more of the following (Milton, 1973):

1. To remove an unsightly blemish.
2. To remove a lesion causing nuisance symptoms, e.g. small haemorrhage or rubbing on clothes.
3. To remove a lesion causing the patient or near relatives genuine anxiety.
4. To forestall the development of malignant degeneration in a benign 'mole', i.e. at site of friction or in danger areas such as the palm, sole or genitalia.
5. To provide the tissue diagnosis of a lesion suspected of being a skin cancer or malignant melanoma.

'Partial' versus 'complete' excision

If the reason for the biopsy comes under the heading of 1 to 4 (above) then a partial biopsy is inadequate. Partial excision of a suspected melanoma is unwise because: (1) malignant degeneration of a benign lesion is often not homogeneous (p. 11) and (2) the treatment of melanoma is influenced by the depth of the tumour, and a histological assessment of this at different parts of the lesion is important in planning treatment and can be obtained by excision biopsy

The only indications for partial biopsy are:

1. A very large pigmented lesion, the removal of which might be grossly disfiguring and may be considered for non-surgical treatment, e.g. a patient with cardiac failure and a pigmented lesion.
2. Any skin lesion for which the definitive treatment is *not* surgical excision, e.g. some squamous cell or basal cell cancers to be treated with radiotherapy.

It used to be believed that partial biopsy increased the risk of spread but this seems unlikely and more cogent reasons against partial biopsy are those given above.

Extent of biopsy

The reason for the biopsy will define its extent. If the lesion is benign and excision is to allay anxiety or to remove a blemish, then the operation will be adequate if the whole of the visible lesion is removed and 2 mm or so of normal tissue around it will include any microscopic extensions. If the lesion is to be treated by radiotherapy and consequently a partial biopsy is desirable, the size of the biopsy must meet the requirements of the pathologist responsible for the diagnosis. Small punch biopsies must avoid the necrotic centre of the tumour, or taking so much normal skin that the tumour gets 'lost' when the sections are cut. A larger wedge biopsy may include a small amount of normal skin but the tumour near its edge is most likely to provide the diagnosis.

If the lesion is thought to be a malignant melanoma and the biopsy is for a tissue diagnosis, the excision is a diagnostic test and not a therapeutic procedure. It is important to make the distinction because, for diagnosis, the lesion, the whole lesion and practically nothing but the lesion is all that is required. A therapeutic excision is often extensive, and because malignant melanoma frequently recurs in operation wounds, it is desirable that the two operative fields do not transgress each other. Any attempt to achieve the best of both worlds by enlarging the diagnostic excision and shrinking the therapeutic one may be dangerous and encourage local recurrence.

Timing

Any patient with malignant melanoma is in danger and it is difficult to prove whether this is increased by a time interval between the diagnostic and therapeutic excisions. If the biopsy excision is assumed to be therapeutic and no further treatment is undertaken until a recurrence develops in the scar, then the prognosis is bad. However, a short delay between diagnostic and therapeutic excisions does not, in my experience, appear to affect the prognosis.

Two operations will be described. In one the lesion is presumed to be benign and is being removed to allay anxiety. In the other, the lesion is presumed to be a malignant melanoma and the biopsy is for tissue diagnosis and immediate therapeutic surgery is contemplated.

Excision of a benign lesion

The surgeon is presumed to be operating on his own without a scrubbed assistant and with limited equipment. Premedication is unnecessary for the majority of patients. Every step of the preparation and the injection of local anaesthetic must be explained and the patient reassured that after the insertion of the local anaesthetic he may feel some 'pressure' but no pain. The skin is prepared from the lesion to a radius of about 10 cm. If the lesion is near the eyes, the patient should hold a sterile swab over them. If the lesion is on the hand or forearm, the easiest skin preparation is for the patient to wash his hands like a surgical scrub and leave them wet. The area is then draped.

The local anaesthetic used is 1 per cent lignocaine with adrenaline (1:200 000), and an intradermal weal is raised in the line of the proposed incision (26 gauge, 2·5 cm needle) and about 2 diameters from the edge of the lesion. As the lesion is benign it is unnecessary to spread the local anaesthetic over a wide area, so the next step is to take a 3·8 cm (21 gauge) needle and inject 1–5 ml into the superficial layers of the dermis, beneath and close to the lesion (Fig. 2.4).

Two frequent errors are made when infiltrating local anaesthetic; either it is placed too deeply, or insufficient time is allowed for it to take effect. If the patient feels any pain during the procedure, the anaesthetic has been placed incorrectly. The depth of infiltration for benign lesions is better assessed by touch than appearance. As the needle is inserted beneath the lesion, place the index finger of the left hand over the point of the needle. As the anaesthetic is injected it can be felt distending the superficial dermis. If a definite swelling is not felt after about $\frac{1}{4}$–$\frac{1}{2}$ ml has been injected, either the needle is too deep or its tip is in a vein (very rare); in either event, reposition the needle. If the injection is made in the superficial part of the dermis, the skin develops an 'orange skin'

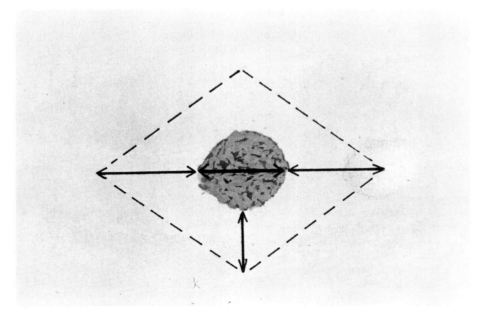

Fig. 2.4   Diagram showing the position for insertion of local anaesthetic for excision biopsy of a presumed benign lesion.

appearance, while injection at slightly deeper levels causes the lesion to stand up on a mound. If the lesion is on the sole or palm it may hurt to shove a needle through the thick skin. This can be avoided by raising a weal of anaesthetic on either side of the dorsum of the foot (hand) and pass a long needle to lie beneath the skin to be anaesthetised. *N.B.:* Adrenaline should never be used in digital nerve blocks.

The shape of the incision, like the upper dashed line in Figure 2.5, will leave no 'dog ears' provided the incision can be at least 3 to 4 times the diameter of the skin to be excised. The elliptical incision is shorter but is apt to leave 'dog ears'. The long axis of these incisions is placed in Langer's line or the most convenient direction. The line in the lower diagram is used only on rare occasions where the lesion is not easily seen and the patient does not want to have rotation or advancement flaps (e.g. a lesion covered by hair in the scalp). Hueston (1973) has described a useful and simple Z-closure which diminishes tension of skin wounds (Fig. 2.6).

The incision is made through the superficial layers of the skin in such a way that the whole incision is marked out with a knife before the full skin thickness has been divided (Fig. 2.7).

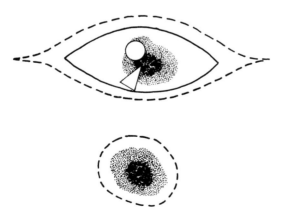

Fig. 2.5   Shows the various biopsy incisions described in the text. The sites for partial biopsy are shown by the clear circle (punch) and clear triangle (wedge biopsy). Note for each of these the necrotic centre of the tumour must be avoided and the site should include the actively growing portion of the tumour.

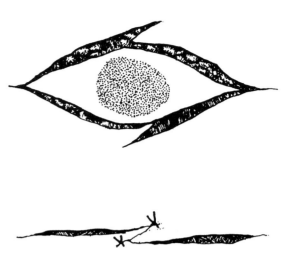

Fig. 2.6   Shows a Z-plasty as described by Hueston (1973) for small excisions.

This step is useful because if the incision is deepened on one side prior to completing it on the other, elasticity of the skin will distort the area and make the second side of the incision difficult to complete accurately. The incisions are deepened and completed with a size 15 blade, by holding the normal tissue just wide of the lesion with a skin hook and working first along one side and then the other (Fig. 2.8). Any pulsating bleeding points are underrun with a catgut stitch-tie. The defect is best closed without tension on the superficial parts of the skin. This is achieved by approximating the dermis and subcutaneous tissues with a 3/0 or 4/0 chromic catgut stitch passed from the deep to the superficial aspect of the wound edge and across the wound (Fig. 2.9). This places the knot in the depths of the wound so that the cut ends do not protrude. The skin is apposed with fine 3/0 or 5/0 and these are inserted as mattress sutures or through and through sutures down to the dermo-epidermal junction (Fig. 2.10).

The wound is sealed with a plastic spray or Friar's Balsam (Tinct. Benz Co). The patient is asked to keep the area dry for 48 hours, to report any undue discomfort, and to avoid knocking the area. The sutures are removed in 7 to 10 days, except in sites where the skin may be inadvertently stretched and the wound torn

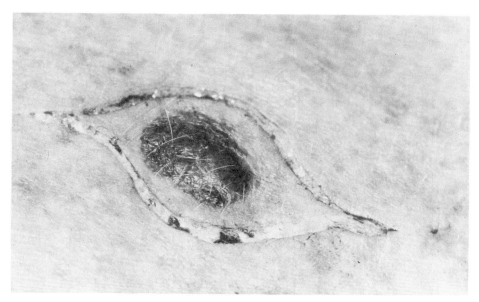

Fig. 2.7   Shows an incision around both sides of the lesion but not made deeper than the superficial dermis.

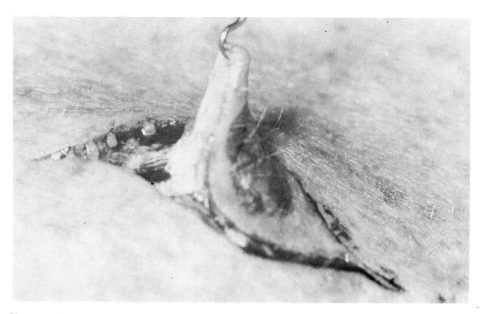

Fig. 2.8   Shows the lesion held up with a skin hook, while the excision is completed close to the surface of the lesion in the subcutaneous fat.

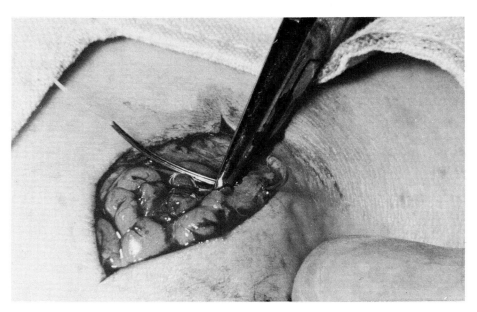

Fig. 2.9   The 4/0 chromic catgut suture has been partly inserted. The stitch enters the subcutaneous fat from the deep aspect, at the upper edge of the wound and emerges just under the skin then passes across the wound to be inserted from the superficial deep plane.

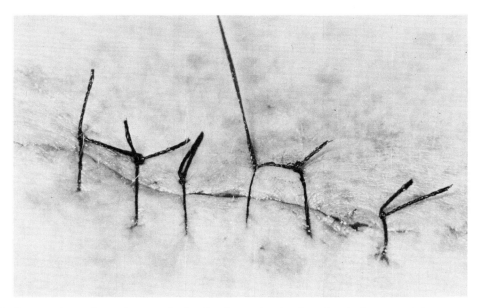

Fig. 2.10   Because the strain on the wound edges has been taken by the subcuticular catgut it is unnecessary to use thick suture material to close the wound and either adhesive stitches or 5/0 black silk is usually adequate except for sites where the skin is particularly thick, such as the sole of the foot.

open, in which case some stitches are left in place for two weeks.

There are some minor modifications to the above technique in special sites:

1. If the lesion is on the back, slightly stronger suture material may be needed as the skin is thicker here than elsewhere. It is also wise to leave the skin stitches in a few days longer on the back than in other sites.

2. Closure of biopsy wounds on the face and neck should be accomplished with the finest sutures (e.g. 5/0) or adhesive stitches. The scar of the stitches about the face can also be reduced by removing them early, e.g. in a few days, and protecting the wound by transverse strapping.

3. In elderly people it is wise to assess carefully the blood supply to the feet before carrying out any biopsy (or other surgery). A pulseless, cold foot, once cut may never heal.

Biopsy for a lesion presumed to be malignant melanoma

The 'line of spread' from the site of the primary lesion to the nearest draining lymph nodes is marked out; this may be difficult if the lesion is near a watershed. However, the main direct course to one or more lymph gland areas is marked. The line of the skin incision for the biopsy should be a direct extension of this line of spread. The operation then follows a similar path to that done previously.

If a frozen section examination is available and the surgeon plans to continue with a definitive operation for melanoma, the biopsy technique is modified in the following ways:

1. The patient has a general anaesthetic.

2. After completing the excision close to the edge of the lesion and after bleeding has been stopped, the wound is filled with a small fragment of gauze swab saturated in 1 per cent Cetavlon and the wound is closed over this with a continuous stitch of 3/0 atraumatic black silk in an attempt to make the wound watertight. The wound is then covered with a dry gauze and a piece of Steridrape* or similar material in order to diminish seeding cells from the wound. One per cent Cetavlon has been shown by Stephens (1969) to be effective in preventing the seeding of cancer cells into wounds.

3. If the pathology report confirms malignancy then the operation for therapeutic excision is carried out in such a way that the field of the diagnostic and therapeutic excisions do not cross one another. If the diagnosis is not confirmed, the small wound is undone, the gauze removed and the wound closed in the usual way.

If the biopsy of a suspected melanoma is done when there is no intention of continuing to the therapeutic excision at the same operation, the direction of the incision and the depth of the excision is the same as described but the wound is closed in the ordinary way and allowed to heal before the formal therapeutic excision is carried out.

Several non-biopsy methods for establishing the diagnosis of malignant melanoma have been assessed in the Melanoma Clinic, but all have been found either unreliable or imprecise when measured against the accuracy of a good biopsy. These methods include thermography, cytology of the surface, electrical conductivity and uptake of radioactive P_{32}.

REFERENCES

Clark, W. H. Jr, From, L., Bernadino, E. A., *et al.* (1969) The histogenesis and biologic behaviour of primary human malignant melanoma of the skin. *Cancer Research*, **29**, 705.
Hueston, J. T. (1973) Z-Closure. *Medical Journal of Australia*, **1**, 496.
Hutchinson, J. (1892) Senile freckles. *Archives of Surgery*, **3**, 319.
Hutchinson, J. (1894) Lentigo melanosis. A further report. *Archives of Surgery*, **5**, 252.
Hutchinson, J. (1896) Pigmentation of the lips and mouth: a case demonstrated by Dixon at the Clinical Museum. *Archives of Surgery*, **7**, 290.

* Manufactured by the 3M Company.

Jacobs, J. B., Edelstein, L. M., Snyder, L. M., *et al.* (1975) Ultrastructural evidence for destruction in the halo nevus. *Cancer Research*, **35,** 352.

Lever, W. F. (1961) *Histopathology of the Skin.* 3rd edition, pp. 415 & 531. Philadelphia: Lippincott.

McGovern, V. J. & Lane Brown, M. M. (1969) *The Nature of Melanoma.* A: p. 94; B: p. 69; C: p. 109; D: p. 95; E: p. 96; F: p. 156; G: p. 87. Springfield: Thomas.

McGovern, V. J., Milton, G. W. & Maxwell, G. A. *Multiple Primary Melanoma* (in press).

Milton, G. W., Lane-Brown, M. M. & Gilder, Mary (1967) Malignant melanoma with an occult primary lesion. *British Journal of Surgery*, **54,** 651.

Molesworth, J. (1965) Personal communication.

Spitz, S. (1948) Melanomas of childhood. *American Journal of Pathology*, **24,** 591.

Stephens, F. O. (1969) A study of method of improving results of surgical management of potentially curable malignant tumours. M.D. Thesis: submitted to the University of Sydney, New South Wales.

3. Introduction to Treatment

There are many difficulties in measuring the effect of surgical treatment, and it is partly because of these that the discussion continues about the most prudent method of treating patients with malignant melanoma. One factor which makes it difficult to establish the correct treatment is that the same word can have many meanings. The following is a brief list of the main terms which cause these problems:

DIAGNOSIS

Has the diagnosis been established by clinical or histological criteria? Clinical assessment even by the most experienced is not sufficiently accurate to be the sole method of establishing the diagnosis.

INVOLVEMENT OF LYMPH NODES

Early detection of involvement of lymph nodes will depend on the skill of the clinician. Hence staging of the disease based solely on the clinical examination of the lymph nodes may vary in different clinics. Pathological involvement of lymph nodes will depend partly on the technique used to carry out the pathological examination. A random section of lymph nodes will give a much lower positive node count than will serial sections of every node removed.

WIDE RESECTION

To many surgeons wide resection means complete excision of macroscopic tumour and a small margin of normal skin; to others wide resection may include extensive and measured skin excision down to and including the deep fascia.

RADICAL DISSECTION OF LYMPH NODES

This is the hardest operation of all to define, because a reliable test for completeness of lymph node excision is either difficult to devise or too elaborate for routine use. So the surgeon who removes lymph nodes for malignancy does not have an available test for completeness of his surgery in the same way that a Hollander insulin test detects the incompleteness of vagotomy. I surmise that 'radical dissection' of lymph nodes means different operations to different surgeons. This opinion is the result of seeing many patients with recurrent melanoma in lymph node areas that have allegedly been cleared of nodes by radical surgery.

DEEP FASCIA

On the limbs and neck the deep fascia is an easily identified tissue with an usually clear line of separation between it and the muscles beneath. Excision of the deep fascia is therefore a precise statement of a definite part of an operation, when used in relation to excision on the limbs. However, even on the limbs there are sites in which either the deep fascia forms part of the muscle attachment, e.g. the upper tibialis anterior muscle, or the fascia merges with the subadjacent tissue plane, e.g. the periosteum of the anterior-medial aspect of the tibia. On the trunk, there is no true deep fascia similar to that found on the limbs (Grant Boileau and Basmajian, 1965). The superficial fascia of the trunk merges with the perimysium of the muscles and may form a discrete layer which can easily be dissected off the muscle (e.g. over the latissimus dorsi muscle). However, as on the limbs there are places where this layer forms part of the muscle attachment and fuses with the muscle and portion of the adjacent bones, e.g. the infraspinatus and the spine of the scapula. In the present account, excision of the deep fascia on the limbs means what it says where applicable; on the trunk excision includes the perimysium of the muscles in the region if it could be separated from them, but not if removal would have been traumatic to the muscle.

The term 5-year survival is accepted by tradition as a satisfactory measure of the success of cancer treatments and it has the advantage of being simple and precise. However, the duration of life has a value—which of us would not choose to have 4 years of useful life rather than, say, $2\frac{1}{2}$? Hence a procedure which allows a patient a year or more of healthy life may be justified while not appearing satisfactory in 5-year survival figures. The problem is further complicated by the concept of the quality of life. It is easy enough to describe life of either excellent or bad quality, but it is hard to measure this in numbers. Suppose two patients each have a malignant melanoma excised and each die about four years later from cerebral metastasis. The first patient lives a full life, apparently free of disease until a few months before his death, the second develops local or intransit recurrences of the disease 18 months after the first treatment and has to be readmitted to hospital on many occasions. The second patient then not only endures repeated treatment, but has the mental strain of seeing his own body diseased. Both patients appear the same on survival statistics.

There are two main schools of thought regarding the treatment of malignant melanoma. One suggests that the most satisfactory treatment is minimal treatment and rely on defence mechanisms of the host to prevent dissemination. The other suggests more and more radical surgery in the hope that this will cure the patient.

As so often happens in discussion probably the more reasonable approach is to try to strike a compromise and devise a method of treatment which will reduce local recurrence to a minimum, reduce the morbidity and mortality to a minimum and interfere as little as possible with the host's defences. The surgeon's difficulty when concerned with such an ideal stems from three factors:

1. He does not yet know to what extent injury, as in a surgical operation, depresses the immune system in the host, i.e. if the draining lymph nodes to a melanoma are excised does this seriously alter the immune mechanisms which prevent dissemination of tumour? There has been much discussion on this subject, but proof in man is not easily obtainable. A dogmatically stated opinion is not always correct.

2. The surgeon is in difficulty when he seeks help from other methods of treatment for melanoma. Radiotherapy may be the treatment of choice for Hutchinson's melanotic freckle (p. 72), but other forms of melanoma, particularly metastases, are often resistant to irradiation. Similarly, chemotherapy in all its forms and hormonal therapy are weak struts to lean on if the patient is potentially curable. The value of immune therapy in preventing or curing generalised spread of melanoma is still not established.

3. Melanoma is undoubtedly a dangerous disease and one which affects people in the prime of life. Chapter 9 will go into some detail on the wide variety of methods we have used for many years in the treatment of incurable melanoma, and it will be seen that sometimes these methods appear to cause a gratifying improvement, but overall the results of treating established metastases are poor.

It is important, I believe, not to suppose that every change is necessarily beneficial. Until a better understanding of the inter-relationship between host and tumour is available it may be wise to be cautious before abandoning careful and thorough surgery. In the final analysis there are only two factors that justify or fail to justify any surgical operation for cancer:

1. The number of patients and the duration of their survival treated surgically as opposed to those treated by other means.

2. The morbidity and mortality of the treatment and of the disease.

The main tenets held by the author in planning treatment are:

1. The treatment of malignant melanoma depends on several factors and there is no hard and fast rule.

2. If surgical ablation of lymph node

drainage area is to be carried out at all, it should be done as thoroughly as possible.

3. The *line of spread* concept, originally proposed by Handley (1906, 1907), is useful in designing surgical treatment. My experience does not accord with the suggestion that cutaneous melanoma develops in a potentially malignant field of susceptible skin for the following reasons: (a) recurrent tumours tend to lie along the line of spread; (b) multiple primary tumours are comparatively rare and do not often lie close to one another.

4. Although it is interesting and may be instructive to find unsuspected tumour deposits in excised lymph nodes, the pathology report is not crucial in justifying or failing to justify surgical treatment. Survival and the quality of survival is the only yardstick.

5. No ablative surgery is contemplated until a firm tissue diagnosis has been established in all cases.

6. At nearly all stages of the disease some therapeutic manœuvres are justified. This includes those manœuvres which are done for the relief of mental or physical distress of patients with terminal disease (see Ch. 13).

7. It is the surgeon's responsibility to maintain a personal interest in his patients until the patient dies. As a corollary of this, in the apparently successfully treated patient the follow-up is as much an integral part of the surgery as the operation itself, and in those patients who die the interest shown by the surgeon has an important part to play in the emotional management of advanced malignancy.

Meticulous follow-up of the patient in the first three years after definitive resection is crucial because potentially curable recurrence of the melanoma is more frequent at this time than in later years (pp. 53 and 75).

The routine follow-up at this clinic is:

a. The patient reports once a month for 18 months and once every second month for another 18 months.

b. At each visit, apart from general enquiries about the patient's health, all likely sites for local recurrence are carefully examined.

c. The patient is asked to report immediately if he feels a lump.

d. After three years the patient is asked to report near each anniversary of the operation.

Treatment

The surgical treatment of malignant melanoma depends on:

1. The wishes of the patient after a careful explanation of the disease and the reasons for treatment (see Appendix to this chapter).

2. The age, sex and general condition of the patient.

3. The site and extent of the disease. The extent includes the depth of penetration of the primary tumour together with any evidence of spread and the extent of this dissemination.

SEX, AGE AND GENERAL CONDITION OF THE PATIENT

This affects the treatment in a variety of ways. The reason for the sex difference in the behaviour of melanoma is not understood; however, melanoma is more dangerous in men than in women (p. 75).

Age and general health can be bracketed together under the heading of 'life expectancy of the patient'. If, melanoma apart, the patient has a life expectancy of 10 years or more, then thorough ablative surgery can be justified on the anticipated benefits for the patient, provided the other factors mentioned below are taken into account. If the life expectancy is less than 10 years, due to either age or debilitating disease, then the possible advantages of ablative surgery are less apparent. Age probably does not have a profound effect on the degree of malignancy of the tumour.

TYPE, SITE AND EXTENT OF THE DISEASE

Malignant melanoma arising in a Hutchinson's melanotic freckle is not likely to spread beyond the site of origin (McGovern, 1952) and extensive removal of lymph nodes is not indicated (p. 11).

The significance of the site of a nodular melanoma affects the choice of treatment in two ways.

1. The situation of the tumour may determine the type or extent of surgery feasible without excessive morbidity, e.g. the amputation of a toe may cause little morbidity while extensive surgery about the face could be very mutilating.

2. The prognosis is affected by the site in some instances, e.g. lymph node involvement is more likely with a primary lesion on the trunk than with a lesion on the limbs (Veronesi *et al.*, 1972; Veronesi, Cascinelli and Preda, 1971).

The size of the primary tumour influencing the prognosis may be assessed in two ways—clinical and pathological. The diameter of the lesion alone does not appear to affect the chance of lymph node metastases (Veronesi *et al.*, 1972; Veronesi, Cascinelli and Preda, 1971). However, the depth of penetration is more significant to the outcome and is related to the elevation of the surface of the tumour above the surrounding skin (Little, 1972). From a clinical assessment, therefore, it appears that the most dangerous lesion is raised or pedunculated. The depth of penetration as assessed microscopically has been shown many times to be related to both the chance of spread and the chance of survival (Beardmore, Quinn and Little, 1970; Allen and Spitz, 1953; McLeod *et al.*, 1968; McLeod *et al.*, 1971; Cochran, 1968; Cochran, 1969a; Cochran, 1969b; Petersen, Bodenham and Lloyd, 1962; Clark *et al.*, 1969; Breslow, 1970; Mehnert and Heard, 1965; McGovern, 1970; Jones, Williams *et al.*, 1968; and Wright, 1949).

The clinical assessment of involvement of lymph nodes is difficult at a stage when it is important to make the diagnosis, because many patients are young, thin and have often had a biopsy of the primary lesion and so the draining nodes are palpable in more than 50 per cent; however, this does not mean the nodes are invaded by tumour.

Irrefutable evidence of systemic spread of the disease immediately alters the whole philosophy of treatment which then becomes centred on palliative or investigative methods (p. 89).

    * Sandoz.

GENERAL PRINCIPLES OF OPERATIONS

1. Hypotensive anaesthesia is advantageous as it considerably reduces blood loss.

2. Diathermy is controlled and used by the first assistant, who has a pair of Riches insulated forceps (Downs Catalogue No. F226). The assistant will seal all small blood vessels, if possible, before they are divided.

3. The donor site of a skin graft is cared for as follows:

The skin is taken to a thickness of 0·3 mm and the raw area covered for up to half an hour with a gauze swab saturated with POR 8 1 ml in 50*. The gauze is then replaced with a thick greasy dressing (3 layers of Jellonet) firmly held in place by dressing pads and crêpe bandages. Donor site is left undisturbed for two, preferably three weeks. The patient can shower by covering it with a plastic sheet. The only indication for taking the dressing down is infection beneath it. If the dressings become adherent to the donor site, the outer bandages are removed and the patient sits in a warm bath for up to three-quarters of an hour before the deeper layers are removed.

APPENDIX

INFORMATION FOR PATIENTS RELATING TO MALIGNANT MELANOMA

Compiled by the staff of the Melanoma Unit, Sydney Hospital

Malignant melanoma is a curable form of skin cancer, although if you read books or articles on the subject written overseas, it is often suggested that the disease is incurable. This idea does not apply in Australia and the reason will be explained later on.

The skin is a complicated organ and not simply a protective sheet; it is made up of many different kinds of cells each having their own special function. The cells responsible for producing suntan also produce many forms of birthmark such as a 'mole' or a freckle, as well as malignant melanoma. These cells are called 'melanocytes', a word which comes from the Greek and means: 'melano'—black and 'cytes'—cells; hence 'the black cells'. They are so called because they produce a secretion which in its concentrated form is jet black. Normally this secretion is spread into many other cells in the skin in such a way that it will produce a brown protective colour (this is suntan) which shields the tissues against strong sunlight.

Usually the melanocytes are spread evenly in the deeper layers of the skin, but it is common for the skin to be slightly badly formed in some areas. These malformations are sometimes present at birth or more often develop in early childhood. They are usually called 'moles', although doctors give them a variety of names depending on the type. The common medical family name for a mole is 'naevus'.

The enormous majority of moles are harmless and remain so throughout life and it is unlikely that more than one in a million will ever produce a cancer. If it does, that cancer is known as a malignant melanoma. The word malignant means that the growth is capable of spreading to other parts of the body. Malignant does *not* mean that the growth *has* spread or that it always *will* spread; it means only that it is *capable* of doing so. A benign growth by its nature is unable to spread beyond the tissue from which it arose.

The first sign of malignant melanoma noticed by the patient is a mole or a birthmark which enlarges and this may be either a flat spreading stain around the mole or a mole which used to be flat becoming raised and lumpy. The mole also becomes darker brown or black. Occasionally, for reasons that are not understood, it may become flesh coloured, i.e. pink. Another change noticed by the patient is that the mole may bleed a little after it is rubbed with clothing, or it may itch. The itch is not severe and it usually comes and goes. As a rule these changes, particularly the growth and the colour change, are noticed by the patient for a period of a few months.

A change that comes on so gradually that you think the mole has been altering for some years is very unlikely to be malignant because malignant growth is always rapid, e.g. it develops in 3 to 12 months.

All moles or naevi tend to change slightly at two periods during life. One at puberty when it is common for moles to enlarge and get darker, and the other during pregnancy when the same thing happens. Therefore, the thing to watch for in a mole is a fairly rapid change developing over a period of months.

Malignant melanoma is rarely painful. The danger of a malignant melanoma is that it will spread and it usually spreads first to the lymph glands. These are small collections of glands situated in the groin, the armpit and the neck which act as filters for any infection or cancer which develops in the tissues; if a melanoma starts to spread, the cells are usually trapped in these lymph glands before the disease spreads further.

In the early stages when the tumour has first reached the lymph glands, there is no way of detecting its presence. However, it is possible to get a reasonable idea about the risk of spread by measuring with a microscope the depth to which the melanoma has grown under the skin. If the melanoma has grown well under the skin, it is often wise to have the glands removed when the original treatment is carried out. But if the melanoma is close to the surface, there is usually little need to remove the glands because the risk of spread is small.

Removing the glands causes little disability, apart from the scar of the operation, although in the case of the groin there may be some swelling in the leg after the operation. However, both the scar and the swelling can nearly always be concealed by simple rearrangement of clothing.

If the disease is caught early, then adequate treatment can nearly always cure it. Operations, whether they involve removing the glands or not, are not dangerous. Patients may be uncomfortable for a few days after an operation, but it is very unusual for them to have more than temporary discomfort. Most of the operations for malignant melanoma involve some form of skin graft. This is not painful, although the donor site from which the skin is taken (usually the thigh) is often more uncomfortable than the operation site. The reason is that the place from which the skin is taken tends to be rather raw, somewhat like a burn, and this makes it sore. The reason for taking the skin from the thigh is that it is easier to keep a dressing on this area. The dressing is left in place for some two to three weeks, by which time the rawness has gone out of the tissues beneath.

Once the wound has fully healed, which takes a couple of weeks or so, the patient should get back to a perfectly normal life and be only slightly restricted in any activity whether at work or play. Any remaining stiffness in joints near the operation site should have resolved completely within a few months. The amount of time off work following these operations is variable and it is best to ask one of the members of the medical team about this in your particular case. However, as a rule, the patient should be back to work in a month or less.

The object of all surgery for malignant melanoma is to remove all the disease at the first major operation, and this can usually be done. However, if the disease ever does start to recur, there are many new methods of treatment that are frequently successful and new methods still being continually investigated.

From the patients treated at the Melanoma Unit, Sydney Hospital, for a superficial melanoma, i.e. one close to the skin surface, more than 95 per cent of patients are free of disease in five years. If the glands have been involved with tumour, the five-year survival is more than 60 per cent. In nearly all instances the chance of cure is good.

Some further facts about malignant melanoma

1. It is rare. The average general practitioner would not see more than one or two cases a year.

2. It is very rare indeed in children before puberty. The youngest case seen at the Melanoma Unit, Sydney Hospital, was a child of 5 years. However, out of the 1600 patients with malignant melanoma seen at the unit, only six of them were under 10.

3. Although malignant melanoma should be cured by the first operation, it is a sensible precaution for anyone who has been treated for this disease to have a regular check-up for at least three years, because a great deal can be done for recurrent melanoma as long as it is treated quickly.

4. It is important that the person returns to a fully normal life and puts the thoughts of the disease behind him as far as possible.

It is the policy of members of the Melanoma Unit to discuss patient's problems openly and with complete frankness, as we do not believe it is possible that an adult can be satisfactorily treated without his own understanding and co-operation. Accordingly, we will be frank with you and ask that you are in return frank with us and that you will ask members of the Unit questions on matters that are causing you anxiety.

REFERENCES

Allen, A. C. & Spitz, S. (1953) Malignant melanoma; a clinicopathology analysis of the criteria for diagnosis and prognosis. *Cancer*, **6,** 1.
Beardmore, G. L., Quinn, R. L. & Little, J. H. (1970) Malignant melanoma in Queensland: pathology of 105 fatal cutaneous melanomas. *Pathology*, **2,** 277.
Breslow, A. (1970) Thickness, cross-sectional areas and depth of invasion in the prognosis of cutaneous melanoma. *Annals of Surgery*, **172,** 902.
Clark, W. H., Jr, From, L., Bernadino, E. A., *et al.* (1969) The histogenesis and biologic behaviour of primary human malignant melanoma of the skin. *Cancer Research*, **29,** 705.
Cochran, A. J. (1968) Method of assessing prognosis in patients with malignant melanoma. *Lancet*, ii, 1062.
Cochran, A. J. (1969a) Histology and prognosis in malignant melanoma. *The Journal of Pathology*, **97,** 459.
Cochran, A. J. (1969b) Malignant melanoma: A review of 10 years' experience in Glasgow, Scotland. *Cancer*, **23,** 1190.
Grant Boileau, J. C. & Basmajian, J. V. (1965) *A Method of Anatomy.* 7th edition. Baltimore: Williams and Wilkins.
Handley, W. S. (1906) On lymphatic permeation as a factor in the dissemination of melanotic sarcoma with a note on operative treatment. *Archives of the Middlesex Hospital*, 7, 52.
Handley, W. S. (1907) The pathology of melanotic growths in relation to their treatment. *Lancet*, i, 927.

Jones Williams, W., Davies, K., Jones, W. M., *et al.* (1968) Malignant melanoma of the skin; prognostic value of histology in 89 cases. *British Journal of Cancer*, **22**, 452.

Little, J. H. (1972) Histology and prognosis in cutaneous malignant melanoma. In *Melanoma and Skin Cancer. Proceedings of the International Cancer Conference, Sydney, 1972*, ed. McCarthy, W. H., p. 107. Sydney: Government Printer.

McGovern, V. J. (1952) Melanoblastoma. *Medical Journal of Australia*, **1**, 139.

McGovern, V. J. (1970) The classification of melanoma and its relationship with prognosis. *Pathology*, **2**, 85.

McLeod, G. R., Beardmore, G. L., Little, J. H., *et al.* (1971) Results of treatment of 361 patients with malignant melanoma in Queensland. *The Medical Journal of Australia*, **1**, 1211.

McLeod, G. R., Davis, N. C., Herron, J. J., *et al.* (1968) A retrospective survey of 498 patients with malignant melanoma. *Surgery, Gynecology and Obstetrics*, **126**, 99.

Mehnert, J. H. & Heard, J. L. (1965) Staging of malignant melanomas by depth of invasion; a proposed index to prognosis. *American Journal of Surgery*, **110**, 168.

Petersen, N. C., Bodenham, D. C. & Lloyd, O. C. (1962) Malignant melanomas of the skin; a study of the origin, development, aetiology, spread, treatment, and prognosis. *British Journal of Plastic Surgery*, **15**, 49.

Veronesi, U., Cascinelli, N. & Preda, F. (1971) Prognosis of malignant melanoma according to regional metastases. *American Journal of Roentgenology, Radium Therapy and Nuclear Medicine*, **111**, 301.

Veronesi, U., Cascinelli, N., Balzarini, G. P., *et al.* (1972) The treatment of regional node metastases. In *Melanoma and Skin Cancer. Proceedings of the International Cancer Conference, Sydney, 1972*, ed. McCarthy, W. H., p. 417. Sydney: Government Printer.

Wright, C. J. E. (1949) Prognosis in cutaneous and ocular malignant melanoma: study of 222 cases. *Journal of Pathology and Bacteriology*, **61**, 507.

4. Excision of a Primary Malignant Melanoma without Incontinuity Dissection of Lymph Nodes

The dimensions of the excision for primary melanoma will be influenced by the site of the lesion, the age and general condition of the patient and the size and depth of penetration of the lesion. The morbidity, i.e. mainly the appearance and the immediate complication of an operation involving excision of skin and subcutaneous tissues, increases when the operation involves a skin graft repair rather than simple closure of the wound. It follows that in those patients in whom the morbidity and complications of the operation are of major concern, the object of the operation will be to obtain primary closure. A frail or elderly patient (Figs. 4.1 and 4.2) may therefore require an excision closed without grafting in spite of the fact that this may increase the risk of local recurrence. A younger patient in whom recurrent melanoma is to be avoided at all costs will usually require a larger excision than can be closed by simple suture. Once the surgeon is committed to closing the defect with a skin graft, a modest increase in the extent of the excision does little to affect the morbidity or risk of failure of the graft. There is some evidence (Milton, 1966) which suggests that excision close to the edge of the tumour (i.e. requiring a graft of less than 5 cm maximum diameter) increases the risk of local recurrence. Hence, once the decision has been made to excise the lesion too widely for primary closure, the resultant split skin graft is usually quite large. As a general rule, the wounds are closed by split skin grafts rather than large rotation or advancement flaps. The reason is that if a recurrence occurs it can be detected early, while a deeper full thickness flap might conceal it for a longer period. The local recurrence rate in these cases is low (p. 52).

The following is a description of the operation for a primary malignant melanoma on the lower leg. The lesion clinically appears to be superficial, i.e. it is flat, and the patient is a woman; both these features indicate a favourable prognosis so a prophylactic groin dissection is not considered.

The steps of this operation have been partly mentioned in relation to biopsy (p. 35). The main points will be reiterated here.

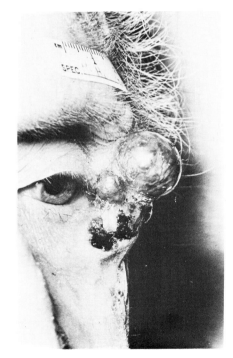

Fig. 4.1 A large fungating malignant melanoma at the outer canthus of the left eye in an 85-year-old woman. The treatment of this lesion consisted of diathermy curettage after establishing the diagnosis by partial biopsy.

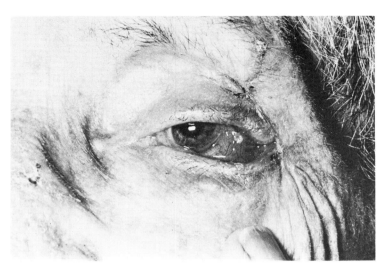

Fig. 4.2   The patient shown in Figure 4.1 three months after operation. The patient lived for nine months after this operation and died of a cerebral haemorrhage.

1. The line of spread is marked out (Fig. 4.3).

2. If the line of spread is not easily determined because the tumour may disseminate in more than one direction, then both lines of spread are marked on the skin and a compromise reached. A primary melanoma near the middle of the posterior aspect of the calf could involve lymphatics in the direction of either the popliteal fossa or those close to the saphenous vein. The excision of such a lesion would therefore be shaped roughly like an inverted triangle, the two long sides of the triangle lying wide of each of the lines of spread.

3. The diagnosis is confirmed by excision biopsy and the wound closed and sealed. The extent of the skin to be removed by the therapeutic excision is marked. The object is to remove 8 to 10 cm of skin along the main lines of spread and about 4 to 5 cm of skin on each side and distal to the lesion (Fig. 4.3). The precise extent of this removal will be influenced by the site of the melanoma. The whole area is covered with a sheet of adhesive plastic. The biopsy site is now excised round the elliptical line drawn surrounding the site of the tumour. At all stages of the excision the knife is held aslant the skin in such a way that the skin is undercut away from the area of the ellipse. The excision is begun proximally and works partially around each side until the deep fascia is reached. This is then divided and the whole of the subcutaneous skin and tissues are removed in one piece over an enlarged area made by undercutting wide of the marked area. Haemostasis is checked and the area of the defect is diminished by inserting a continuous subcuticular skin to muscle stitch (2/0 Dexon) around the circumference of the defect. As this stitch is inserted the needle is constantly directed towards the central area of the ellipse. In this way, the narrowing of the defect is made evenly around the whole circumference of the excised area (Fig. 4.4).

4. A split skin graft is obtained from the opposite limb and applied to the defect.

5. A piece of sterile plastic foam is cut to fit the size of the defect, covered with a layer of Jellonet and held in place with firm crêpe bandages.

6. The wound is dressed six days after operation.

Special points

1. *Cutaneous nerves.* In most situations the position of cutaneous nerves may be disregarded because the overlap by adjacent

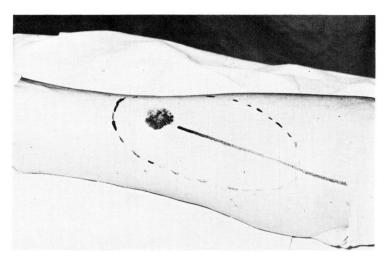

Fig. 4.3 A superficial spreading melanoma on the shin of a middle-aged woman. The line of spread is indicated by the solid line and the extent of excision marked by the dotted line.

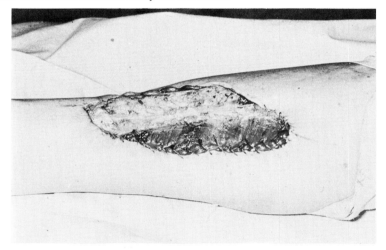

Fig. 4.4 Excision has been completed and the defect somewhat narrowed by a continuous 3/0 Dexon stitch attaching the free skin margin to the underlying muscle. The present technique is to do this with a subcuticular stitch which gives a somewhat neater appearance in the early stages, but here the stitch penetrates the skin.

nerves will compensate for any that are divided. However, major cutaneous nerves can often be preserved. An excision in the mid posterior calf should preserve the sural nerve. The best way to identify such nerves is to seek them, if possible, where they lie beneath the deep fascia in the proximal part of the field and as the dissection proceeds distally follow the nerve with sharp dissection so as to retain the main trunk but not its small branches. Although such a dissection may devascularise the nerve over many centimetres, this does not affect the subsequent function of the nerve.

2. *Undercutting.* The advantages of undercutting the skin in the manner described are two-fold. The skin edge will blend easily with the skin graft without a step between normal subcutaneous tissues surrounding the defect

and the defect itself. The extent of excision of subcutaneous tissues will be increased by undercutting without increasing the defect, and large lymphatics lie about half-way between the skin and deep fascia.

3. In some situations, it is important to adjust the position of the limb *before* the musculo-cutaneous circumferential stitch is inserted. This applies particularly to the back of the calf. The natural position of the foot during much of the excision tends to be plantar-flexed, and if the circumferential stitch is applied while the foot is in this position, it may cause some tearing of the muscle when the ankle is later placed at right angles to the calf.

4. Free grafts on the posterior part of the calf may detach as soon as the patient starts weight-bearing, because there is a tendency for the foot to plantarflex. As soon as the patient walks he applies a shearing strain to the graft area which may be stripped off. The safety of the graft can be assured by making a well-padded plaster back slab before the operation, the patient holding his foot at right angles to the ankle while the plaster sets. On the dorsum of the wrist or forearm, a cock-up splint will ensure adequate immobility of the graft site.

5. In all primary excisions carried out in this series, the deep fascia has been removed as part of the specimen. However, note the difference between 'deep fascia' in different parts of the body (p. 41).

6. Lesions on the back, particularly between the scapulae, may be hard to graft successfully as a primary manœuvre because of the difficulty of maintaining adequate immobility in the early postoperative period. There are three ways of attempting to overcome this difficulty. The patient can be nursed prone. I have not used this technique but patients who have endured it say that after a short time the position becomes most uncomfortable. A second method is to store the skin to be used for the graft in a cold (4°C) Hank's solution for 2 to 3 days. The patient sits out of bed and the skin placed on the defect; no dressings are applied until the evening when the area is dressed and firmly strapped. The graft usually takes with this technique, but there is still the risk that

undue movement may dislodge it. The third method is to place a circumferential purse string of No. 1 black silk about 1 cm wide of the edge of the wound, place the graft in the defect and apply gentle pressure to the graft via a piece of plastic foam held by 3/0 black silk stitch tied across the dressings. This method appears to give the best results in terms of graft take, but there is still a proportion of cases who require a secondary graft. When this method is used it is wise to take the dressings down on the second postoperative day when the patient can sit out of bed. If a portion of the graft is loose, gently irrigate beneath it to remove any serum or blood clot, slit the graft to prevent reaccumulation of serum, and then leave the patient sitting comfortably with the wound exposed and without pressure. A gentle pressure dressing is applied at night and the whole area exposed again each day. We have found that many grafts of doubtful viability will take when exposed in this manner.

7. The appearance of the grafted site can be considerably improved by the correct use of cosmetics, special covering or scar creams and powder. Most of the major cosmetic manufacturers have advisory services which can be of great help to women who are worried by the appearance of the graft.

In summary, it can be said that split skin grafting to defects about the limbs, neck and face and most of the trunk should be followed by nearly 90 to 100 per cent 'take' of the graft, provided the established rules are obeyed. However, some difficulty in obtaining a satisfactory take of a skin graft may be encountered when the defect is between the scapulae.

FOLLOW-UP

The adequate and thorough follow-up of these patients is an integral part of the treatment (p. 43).

Results

Excision of a primary melanoma without lymph node resection was carried out in three circumstances:

1. A superficial primary tumour with negligible penetration into the dermis.

2. Patients who had a short life expectancy

(less than five years) because of ill health or old age.

3. Patients with disseminated disease, when excision of the primary tumour was performed either to establish the diagnosis or to rid the patient of a fungating tumour.

The results of the operation performed at the Clinic will be considered only for those patients who had simple excision (with or without free graft repair) as a definitive operation designed to rid the patient of his disease. In the other two groups, excision of the primary tumour was only the first stage of treatment with chemotherapy or immunetherapy, the results of which are considered in Chapter 9.

Two hundred and fifty-seven patients had a wide excision without lymph node dissection as the definitive treatment for melanoma. Thirty-three of these patients are not considered further for one of four reasons:

1. Twenty-one were lost to follow-up and no record of their deaths can be found.

2. Eight patients died of causes not related to the melanoma. One of these patients had known small secondary deposits of tumour when he died of a coronary occlusion: the other seven were free of all sign of melanoma at death.

3. Four patients had incurable and fungating tumours removed as a palliative procedure.

4. No patient who had an occult primary melanoma is considered here.

The remaining 224 patients had simple excision of the primary ($\pm$ free graft repair) as the definitive treatment for melanoma.

These patients can be subdivided on the basis of the site of the primary tumour in relation to the draining lymph nodes, also on sex (Table 4.1).

There were no postoperative deaths following wide excision of a melanoma. In those patients who had a free graft by the technique described there was only one local recurrence of the disease (i.e. recurrence under the graft or at its edge). Thirty-nine patients had primary closure and no free graft after excision of the melanoma, and of these seven developed recurrent disease and were subsequently treated with either further excision, immune therapy or chemotherapy (p. 84). However, the pattern of recurrence and the fate of the patients are shown in Table 4.2.

The overall survival of patients who had excision of the primary melanoma without lymph node resection is shown in Figures 4.5, 4.6 and 4.7, i.e. 76·1 per cent of patients survived five or more years. However, this figure excludes all patients lost to follow-up or who

Table 4.1 The number of patients (and sex) treated by excision of the primary melanoma alone without node dissection as an initial part of their treatment, subdivided by the site of the primary relative to the lymph drainage from the site

	Men	Women	Total
To cervical nodes	12	26	38
To axillary nodes	40	43	83
To inguinal nodes	18	85	103
Total	70	154	224

Table 4.2 Pattern of recurrent melanoma

Patient	Site of recurrent melanoma	Recurrence at:	Death at:
Mr R. B.	Systemic	31/12	37/12
Mrs E. B.	Local	12/12	42/12
Mrs W. M.	Intransit	51/12	87/12
Mrs J. McH.	Systemic	7/12	13/12
Mr M. P.	Local	6/12	54/12
Mr W. B.	Local and lymph nodes	2/12	18/12
Mr F. K.	Intransit and nodes	6/12	9/12

Note: The follow-up of these patients was complete to 31 December, 1975.

died of intercurrent disease; if these are included in the graph, the survival rate for five or more years after operation is 73·8 per cent.

These figures suggest that wide excision and split skin graft is a reasonable method of treating superficial spreading melanoma. The pattern of recurrence referred to implies that careful follow-up after surgery is still justified.

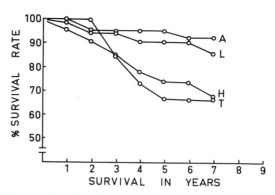

Fig. 4.6 Survival figures for women patients with wide excision and graft alone for malignant melanoma. A = site of primary on the arm; L = on the leg; H = on the head and neck; T = on the trunk.

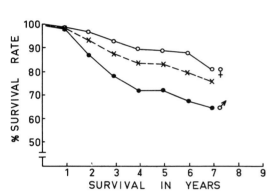

Fig. 4.5 Overall survival figures for wide excision and graft alone.

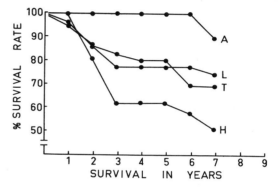

4.7 Survival figures for malignant melanoma treated by wide excision and graft without lymph node dissection for men. A = site of primary on the arm; L = on the leg; T = on the trunk; H = on the head and neck.

REFERENCES

Milton, G. W. (1966) The site and time of recurrence of malignant melanoma. *Medical Journal of Australia*, **1**, 283.

5. Melanoma of the Trunk or Arm

RADICAL DISSECTION OF THE AXILLARY LYMPH NODES

A melanoma situated on the trunk or upper arm could, theoretically, always be treated by an incontinuity excision of the primary lesion and the draining lymph nodes, but there is no need for extensive ablative surgery in every case. A flat, superficial melanoma, especially in a woman, does not require lymphadenectomy because the risk of metastasis is small, although it is none the less wise to follow the patient carefully after local resection in case of unexpected spread (p. 43). Obvious clinical involvement of the nodes is a definite indication for resection, provided the patient's age and general condition are satisfactory. In elderly or frail patients radical lymphadenectomy has also been avoided, and even when the nodes have become clinically involved in such patients, the nodes are treated by direct intranodal injections (p. 89). The indications for dissection of the lymph nodes are given on page 43.

For purposes of this description it is presumed that the patient is a middle-aged man in excellent health who has a lesion on the upper arm having the clinical features of a malignant melanoma. The patient also has a palpable axillary lymph node but it cannot be ascertained whether or not this contains metastatic tumour. The care of this patient falls into the following steps:

Pre-admission preparation

The patient and his wife together discuss the operation with the surgeon; the following points are made by the surgeon:

1. A tissue diagnosis will be established before any radical surgery is done.
2. The patient will be in hospital for approximately 10 days to a fortnight.
3. For two to three months after the operation the patient will have some stiffness of the shoulder particularly in relation to raising the hand above the head. Movements of the hand, wrist and elbow will be unaffected by the operation.
4. If he uses his arm to the full after the operation, his shoulder will return quickly to normal. The best forms of exercise are those which are pleasurable and involve sport, e.g. golf.

Between the time of this visit and the patient's admission to hospital, he is asked to take a daily bath or shower using an antiseptic soap, e.g. Gamophen. The lesion itself is covered with adhesive strapping to protect it from clothing. Chest X-rays are taken and haemoglobin estimated, and immediately prior to operation, two units of blood (1 litre) are reserved for possible transfusion. If the patient is very apprehensive from the time of this interview to the day of the operation, he should be given small quantities of Valium, i.e. 2 mg three times a day and at night, or 5 mg twice a day and at night.

Preoperation preparation in hospital

1. The patient is shaved from the lower half of the neck to the umbilicus, back and front, the complete circumference of one thigh is shaved from the groin to the knee (i.e. the donor site).
2. After the shave, the patient is given a bath using antiseptic soap.

3. One hour before the operation, the patient is given preoperative medication.

The operation

Anaesthesia is induced and the patient is placed supine with the affected arm abducted to 90 degrees and supported on an arm board. The protective strapping on the lesion is removed. The skin is prepared with a standard antiseptic from the neck to the lower ribs, and from the sternum to 5 cm behind the posterior axillary fold. The arm is prepared circumferentially to 5 cm below the elbow. The line of direct spread is drawn from the primary lesion to the centre of the floor of the axilla (Fig. 5.1). The primary lesion is excised close to the macroscopic border of the tumour and the wound sealed as described on page 34. Frozen section examination confirms the diagnosis of melanoma, and the incontinuity radical dissection of the axillary lymph nodes continues. The extent of the skin to be excised is next marked on the skin about 4 cm wide of the line of spread on each side. These skin marks are continued to include the floor of the axilla. Next the incisions required to give total access to the axilla are marked (Fig. 5.2). The main purpose in the design of the operation is to reach the apex of the axilla with the minimum disturbance of the axillary contents and then to carry the dissection from the apex downwards and backwards to the site of the primary tumour following the reverse direction of potential lymphatic tumour spread (Figs. 5.2 and 5.3).

The incisions marked out on the skin indicate two types of incision; those near the line of spread are designed to excise potentially tumour-bearing tissues, while those on the chest wall are to provide access to the axilla. The manner of making the incision is influenced by its purpose. If the object is to excise tumour-bearing tissue, the incision is undercut away from the line of spread in order to excise a wide margin of subcutaneous tissues with the specimen. Incisions designed for access are made at right angles to the surface and the flaps are thick to ensure viability.

Two flaps are raised from the surface of the pectoralis major muscle (Fig. 5.4). The lateral thoracic artery and vein will be found lying close to the free border of the muscle and should be divided between ligatures. A similar lateral flap is of the same thickness and extends laterally until the tendonous portion of the sternal head of the muscle is identified. When this has been done, the groove between the sternal and clavicular heads of the muscle is identified (Fig. 5.4).

The gap between the two parts of the muscle is widened laterally while it is held with small retractors. The small vessels passing between the heads are sealed with the diathermy before division. At the lateral end of the groove will be seen the silvery surface of the anterior aspect of the tendon into which the muscle fibres attach, and this is divided parallel to the humerus and close to the bone from in front. The vessels in the axilla may be protected by a finger passed directly behind the tendon. It is unnecessary to extend the separation of the groove more than about 1 cm medial to the coracoid process, and it is unwise to do so because the lateral pectoral nerve lies close to the undersurface of the muscle. Lift the sternal head of pectoralis major medially as if opening a book (Figs. 5.5 and 5.6). While doing this, divide the small vessels and branches of the median pectoral nerve as they enter the muscle. Next, clear the anterior surface of pectoralis minor until the upper border is defined, then follow the upper border to the coracoid process (Fig. 5.5). Pass a finger behind the muscle as close as possible to the bone and divide the tendon. It is important to keep close to the bone and to identify and preserve the thoracoacromial artery and vein. These lie very close to the medial edge of the extreme upper part of the pectoralis major and their accidental division gives rise to irritating haemorrhage.

Identify the axillary vein by gently pressing the divided medial part of pectoralis minor downwards and medially (Fig. 5.6). Lift the adventitia off the vein and dissect the vein wall free of all areolar tissue. This is done along the anterior surface of the vein until the vein is seen to flatten at its upper limit where it lies on the

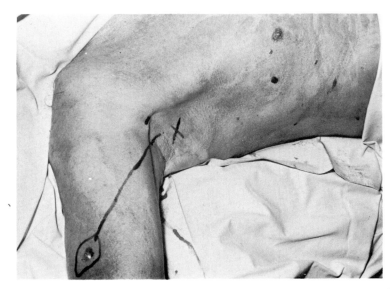

Fig. 5.1   Shows a primary malignant melanoma on the upper arm. The line of spread to the central axilla (x) has been marked, and also the extent of the biopsy excision. Note the latter is in the same axis as the line of spread.

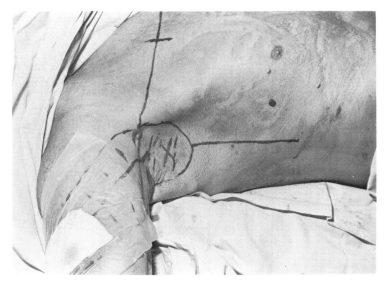

Fig. 5.2   Shows the same patient as in Figure 5.1. The diagnosis has been established and the biopsy wound sealed. The skin to be excised has been marked out (hatched area) and two access incisions have been marked. The anterior of these incisions is drawn on the straight line from the tendon of the pectoralis major to the head of the clavicle.

first rib under the subclavius muscle belly. The tendon of the subclavius arising from the upper surface of the first rib can be seen at the apex of the axilla (Fig. 5.6). The lateral pectoral nerve crosses the vein near this higher level and is preserved.

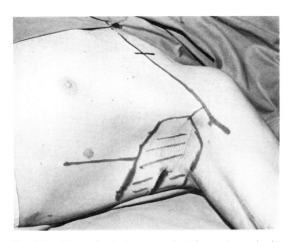

Fig. 5.3 Shows the incisions marked for an incontinuity dissection for a primary melanoma on the back. Note the short incision connecting the axillary resection to the anterior access incision leaves a slightly too long and narrow distal flap from the arm. This error was corrected when the incision was made. All the remaining figures of this operation are of this patient and were taken from approximately the same position.

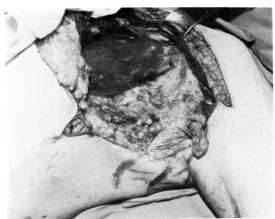

Fig. 5.5 Shows the insertion of the sternal head of the pectoralis major has been divided, folded forwards, and held by an assistant. The pectoralis minor is displayed, while the retractor holds the clavicular head of the pectoralis major out of the way. The lateral pectoral nerve passing to the deep surface of the pectoralis major can be seen taut at the upper border of the pectoralis minor. The medial pectoral nerve passing through the pectoralis minor has been divided.

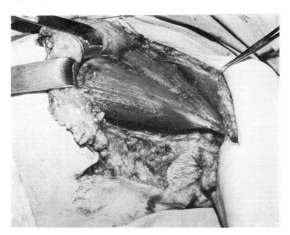

Fig. 5.4 The anterior surface of pectoralis major muscle has been cleared and the groove separating the sternal from the clavicular head can be seen most clearly at the medial end.

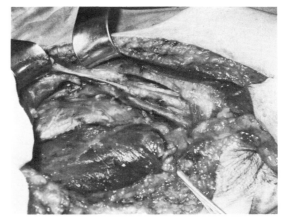

Fig. 5.6 The pectoralis minor has been divided and held downwards with the forceps to display the axillary vessels. Note the lateral thoracic nerve and accompanying vessels held taut by the left retractor. The axillary vein at its upper end has been deflected slightly forwards by the pull of the retractors, but where it curves backwards note the tendon of the subclavius muscle arising from the first rib and passing across the vein.

The formal dissection of the axillary contents now begins at the apex and is achieved by working downwards first on one side and then the other of the adipose tissue in the axilla. The chest wall has no true deep fascia but the areolar tissue forms a well-defined layer and this must be removed with the contents of the axilla by dissecting absolutely flush with the surface of the intercostal muscles. The small branches of the vessels on the chest wall can be sealed by diathermy.

The first big nerve emerging from the chest wall which is accompanied with moderate sized vessels is the lateral division of the second thoracic nerve (the intercostobrachial nerve). The next major nerve encountered is the nerve to serratus anterior. The method of identifying it is to hold the areolar tissue, the axillary contents and the pectoralis minor muscle laterally. The nerve to serratus anterior is then seen through the fascia as a flat white cord which separates from the surface of the serratus with the areola tissue over approximately the middle third of the muscle. The next step is to free the middle third of the nerve from its surrounding fascia. This is done by keeping the tissues slightly on the stretch and using a very sharp scalpel, drawing a line along the edge of the nerve on each side. The nerve is now freed and is followed upwards behind the main axillary vessels. This is done by placing a finger or nerve hook behind the nerve and keeping it taut while sharp dissection proceeds on the edges of the nerve.

Note: It appears from the direction of the nerve that it would be originating from the posterior cord of the brachial plexus, whereas, of course, it originates from C5, 6 and 7 and enters the axilla behind the brachial plexus. However, it is unnecessary to follow the nerve to its origin.

Having identified the nerve as far as the posterior aspect of the axillary vessels, leave the medial wall of the axilla and turn once more to the lateral side, i.e. the axillary vein. This is now thoroughly peeled free of its adventitia while dividing between ligatures all the branches of the vein. As the dissection proceeds from above downwards look for the nerve to latissimus dorsi (Figs. 5.7 and 5.8). This arises from the posterior cord of the brachial plexus and is found by gently pressing the axillary contents medially, when it can be seen near the posterior wall of the axilla diverging downwards slightly from the line of the

axillary vessels. A few small vessels will be seen passing between the posterior aspect of the axillary vessels and subscapularis muscle. These lie behind the fascia on the posterior wall of the axilla and it is unnecessary to divide them as they are posterior to the line of lymph flow. When the upper part of the nerve to latissimus dorsi has been cleared, place a Kocher retractor over the axillary vein and hold it superolaterally. Now demonstrate again the two nerves, one to serratus anterior and the other to latissimus dorsi. In between them will be seen a pyramid of tissues passing behind the main axillary vessel. This contains fat and a few small lymph nodes. By gently dissecting behind this tissue it can be freed and brought forward and the extreme upper limit of it is ligated by passing an aneurysm needle close to the posterior aspect of the main vessels and between the two nerves (Fig. 5.8). An artery forcep is placed on the tissue distal to the ligature and this tissue is then drawn downwards and laterally while the posterior wall of the axilla is cleared from above downwards.

The subscapular vessels are the last major branches of the axillary artery and vein; they are ligated just distal to the point of origin of either the posterior circumflex humeral artery and vein or as high up as convenient. These vessels are then folded downwards with the axillary contents and the circumflex scapular vessels are ligated. While this is being done, the glistening tendon of the latissimus dorsi will be seen just lateral to these vessels (Fig. 5.8). It too must be totally cleared of areolar tissue, the tissues being included with the axillary contents. The nerve to latissimus dorsi is now followed downwards to the point where it enters the muscle and the nerve must be stripped bare by dividing the vessels close to it between artery forceps. It is important to avoid as far as possible getting into the centre of the axilla because dye studies show that lymph vessels may be damaged by doing so. As the nerve to latissimus dorsi approaches the muscle, it usually divides into two branches and either or both of these are easily damaged unless the dissection proceeds from above downwards as described. Division of the nerve does not produce

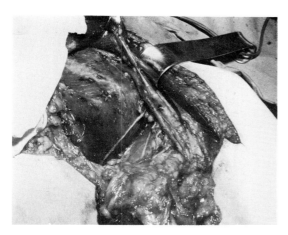

Fig. 5.7 Shows the partly completed dissection. The small dark spots on the chest wall are the marks caused by coagulation of small vessels. The nerves to serratus anterior and latissimus dorsi have been largely cleared. The specimen is reflected posteriorly; it will now be enclosed in thick gauze bandage.

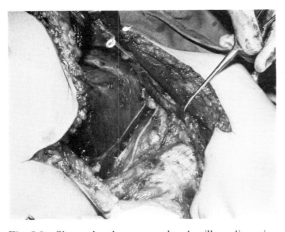

Fig. 5.8 Shows the almost completed axillary dissection. The small blob of fat behind the axillary vessels is the stump of the ligated pyramid of adipose tissue between the two nerves described in the text.

any hardship but it is unnecessary to divide it, unless there are large masses of tumour in the axilla, in which case it may be safer to divide the nerve as Haagensen (1971) suggests.

Now turn to the medial wall of the axilla again and divide the vascular connections between the intercostal vessels and the subscapular vessels flush with the chest wall.

These anastomotic channels number about three to five and they enter or leave the chest wall close to the path of the lower third of the nerve to serratus anterior. The easiest way to deal with them is to pick up the nerve to serratus anterior previously dissected and to pass a finger caudally posterior to the plane of the nerve. By lifting the finger forwards, the anastomotic vessels can be identified and are ligated serially using plain catgut. As each ligature is tied it is important to watch the serratus anterior muscle, and if it twitches the knot must be immediately undone. When all these vessels have been divided and the axillary contents are held laterally, the dissection of the medial wall of the axilla is complete. Test that the nerve to serratus anterior has not been damaged by holding it up by its middle third on a nerve hook and 'blinking' the diathermy electrode on to the handle of the hook, when the muscle will be seen to contract.

The axillary contents are now free of all connections to the walls and remain attached to the floor of the axilla as a pedicle. These contents are now enclosed in a gauze bandage or plastic bag. The remaining incisions are now enlarged in the direction of the tumour site. The knife is held aslant to undercut the skin flaps away from the line of spread.

The first part of the wound to be closed is the axillary dissection as follows:

Abduct and internally rotate the arm on the affected side so that the patient's hand is placed on the lower ribs of the same side. A muscular floor for the axilla is made by lifting the medial border of the tendon of latissimus dorsi forwards with a rake retractor and dividing the medial two-thirds of it parallel and close to the bone. A flap of the medial edge of the muscle can then be lifted forwards. The divided tendon of the pectoralis major is now identified, its upper border is the point to be attached to the side of the clavicular head of the muscle close to its insertion. About two-thirds of the pectoralis major is attached using 2/0 chromic catgut, the distal third being left as a flap to be joined to the border of latissimus dorsi (Figs. 5.9 and 5.10).

Abduct the arm to its former position at right

angles. The skin and subcutaneous wounds on the chest are now closed using 3/0 plain catgut in the fat and 5/0 black silk stitches in those skin wounds that are not under any tension, and 3/0 black silk where the skin is slightly tensed. In the floor of the axilla no attempt is made to oppose the skin edges where the cutaneous floor has been removed but rather

the skin edges of the defect are attached to the muscular curtain of the reconstituted floor with a running subcuticular to muscle Dexon suture (3/0). The black silk stitches are used to reinforce the Dexon and are left long, to be subsequently tied over the dressings on the graft (Figs. 5.11, 5.12 and 5.13).

The patient is now turned over so that the

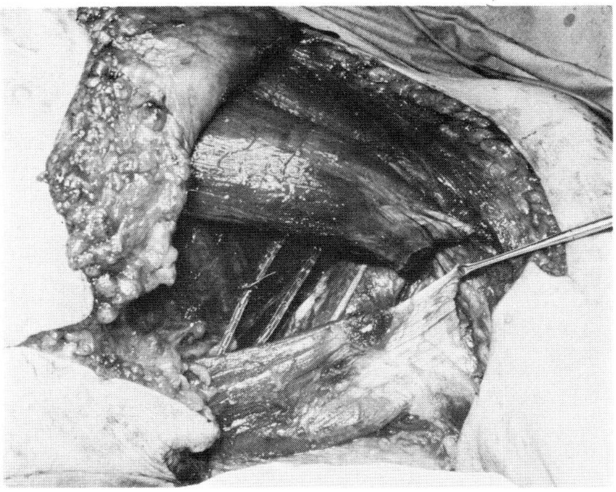

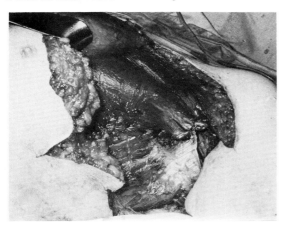

Fig. 5.9   The axillary dissection has been completed. Two small Haemovac drains are held in place on the medial wall with (3/0) plain catgut sutures passed through the superficial parts of the underlying muscle. The insertion of the sternal head of the pectoralis major muscle has been repaired leaving a small portion of the lower border free. The tendon of latissimus dorsi has been partly divided and is held forwards with an Allis forceps.

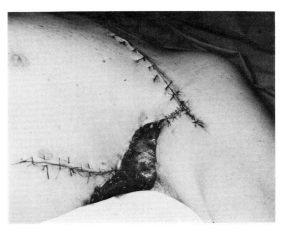

Fig. 5.11   The wounds have been partly closed. The covered specimen still attached by a pedicle is in the lower part of the picture. The subcuticular to muscle Dexon stitch holds the sloping edges of the skin bordering the resected area to the axillary 'floor'.

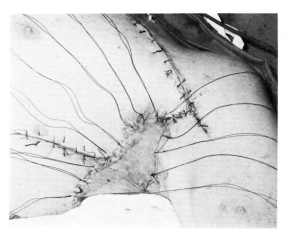

Fig. 5.10   The free borders of pectoralis major and latissimus dorsi have been joined with a running 2/0 chromic catgut stitch, thereby making a muscular curtain floor to the axilla.

Fig. 5.12   A free graft, taken from the thigh, is held in place with interrupted 3/0 black silk stitches which are left long.

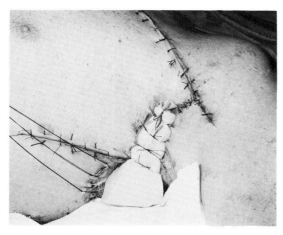

Fig. 5.13 Plastic foam is held firmly against the graft by tying the silk sutures across it in the usual way. The posterior end of the foam is free until the posterior dissection has been completed and the remaining graft fixed in place.

dissection can be completed posteriorly to include the site of the primary tumour and a broad band of skin and subcutaneous tissues en bloc with the axillary contents. The width of the skin resected is approximately 4 cm wide of the line of spread on each side and is undercut a further 1 to 2 cm. The perimysium of the muscles is removed together with the subcutaneous tissues; the defect is closed by a subcuticular to muscle Dexon stitch, and a free skin graft applied in continuity with that in the axillary floor.

Postoperative instructions

1. Penicillin 500 000 units 6-hourly for two days.
2. Check the circulation in the hand on the affected side hourly for the first 12 hours.
3. Be certain of adequate sedation.
4. If suction drains tend to leak so that suction is ineffective, attach the ends of the drain to a continuous suction pump for the first 24 hours.
5. Second day after operation, the patient should be encouraged to sit out of bed for a short time.
6. At each physiotherapy visit the patient should be encouraged to exercise his wrist and hand quite independent of the position of the shoulder, as well as breathing exercises.
7. The dressings are not touched for six days but the patient's comfort will be enhanced if the bandages are taken off after three or four days and immediately reapplied over the dressings. At this stage, the patient can abduct his arm very slightly so that a shoulder spiker bandage can be applied which allows him limited shoulder movement. The suction drains are removed with the first dressing.
8. See page 44 for care of the donor site.

Complications

LOCAL

1. *Shoulder movements*

Initially, shoulder movements are restricted, particularly abduction and external rotation. The enthusiastic patient should have normal shoulder movements within a couple of months, but the rate of recovery will depend on his determination. The patient should be encouraged to use his arm as much as possible and to play all manner of sport. Golf is ideal for improving shoulder movements because the patient can start by putting, then short chip shots, and by the time he has graduated to hitting a drive his shoulder will be normal. The non-sportsman who has little time or inclination for such frivolities should be encouraged to use his arm for all ordinary tasks. Physiotherapy will help to get the shoulder movements started but rapid improvement only comes with the patient's own efforts.

2. *Lymphoedema*

Nearly all patients will develop some lymphoedema of the arm, but this virtually never causes serious disability, unlike leg oedema after groin dissection. The oedema is not usually detectable in the hand, just discernible in the forearm and fairly easily felt in the back of the upper arm. The lymphoedema is very rarely as severe after this operation for melanoma as it can be after radical mastectomy and radiation for carcinoma of the breast.

Streptococcal lymphangitis occasionally develops in the arm any time up to six months after operation. The first symptom of lymphangitis is a rigor which within hours is followed by pain and tenderness in the arm and on the chest wall. The affected arm, hand and chest wall is also swollen and often red and tender to touch. Treatment consists of large doses of penicillin which must be continued for at least a month or the infection is likely to recur.

3. *Failed graft*

If the haemostasis has been satisfactory and the bandages correctly applied there should be no failure of a split skin graft on the arm due to either movement or haematoma. However, if the graft has failed it is as well to strip off all the dead tissue as soon as it is recognised and prepare the wound for a secondary graft if a large area remains, or wait for healing by secondary intention if the defect is small.

4. *Sinus into the axilla*

This is an uncommon complication which may be the result of retained suture material or simply a delay in closing the cavity. It should be managed by irrigating the sinus occasionally and making sure that the patient continues to exercise his shoulder. Any attempt to heal the sinus by immobility of the shoulder will result in prolonged stiffness of the joint.

5. *Sloughing of the skin flaps*

This should be a rare complication and the only one to slough in this series has been a long flap raised on the medial wall of the axilla, the extent of the slough was small (i.e. about 1 cm in diameter). If this occurs the necrotic skin is best excised and the defect either grafted with a split skin graft or left to heal by secondary intention when the patient has returned home and continues shoulder movements.

6. *Numbness*

The patient will invariably notice the inside of his upper arm is numb. This is the result of the division of the intercostobrachial nerve. The patient may be assured that he will cease to notice the numbness in less than 2 to 3 months.

Systemic complications of this operation are rare because the patient can be mobile early in the postoperative period and abdominal respiration is not interfered with.

Notes

The operation described contains many features which have been described before and have been accepted into standard surgical practice, but the procedure has been given from beginning to end for the sake of continuity.

The anaesthetic technique used in these operations follows the standard pattern administered by trained anaesthetists, but the blood loss can be considerably reduced by hypotensive agents during dissection. The volume of bleeding does not appear to be materially reduced unless the systolic blood pressure is below 90 mmHg. The practice used here, in suitable cases, has been to maintain the systolic pressure at between 80 to 90 mmHg during the dissection permitting it to rise to 100 mmHg near the end of dissection before the wounds are closed. This permits the final check of haemostasis to be carried out with a systolic pressure of 100 mmHg or more. Hypotension is not used on any patient who is over 60 years of age or who has had any history suggesting any form of vascular disease.

The average blood loss for these procedures is difficult to determine because although the blood loss in terms of swab weight has been recorded in all patients, the magnitude of the loss is determined by the site of the primary and hence the extent of the dissection of subcutaneous tissue after the axillary dissection has been completed. The average blood loss during the axillary dissection alone is about 350 ml by swab weight and therefore does not usually require replacement by blood, as it constitutes less than a blood donation. However, if extensive dissection has to be carried out across the back the patient may require blood transfusion.

The technique of fashioning a muscular floor to the axilla is required only if it appears necessary to carry a skin graft into this region. This applies particularly when the lesion is situated on the back because the greatest restriction of shoulder movements is produced by a tight posterior axillary fold, and this can be avoided by taking the skin graft into the axilla from behind. Shoulder movements will not be inhibited if most of the dissection is from the front when the lesion is on the anterior chest wall.

Recurrence of melanoma in the axilla is rare following the procedure described here, i.e. less that 5 per cent.

Results

The survival figures for the procedure described are given at the end of Chapter 7, page 75, where they are compared with other lymph node dissections.

REFERENCE

Haagensen, C. D. (1971) *Diseases of the Breast*. 2nd edition. Philadelphia: Saunders.

6. Melanoma of the Lower Trunk and Legs

RADICAL DISSECTION OF THE ILIOINGUINAL LYMPH NODES

The aim of this chapter is to describe the technique of ilio-inguinal lymphadenectomy as it has been performed for melanoma in the watershed of these nodes. The indications for node resection are similar to those for axillary node excision, that is:

1. Obvious clinical involvement of the nodes.
2. Deeply penetrating primary tumour (i.e. into the lower dermis).
3. Pedunculated melanoma.
4. The majority of melanoma in the drainage area in men (except those patients who are frail and elderly or lesions which are entirely superficial with no dermal component).

Technique

Assessment and preparation of the patient follows the same pattern as for other major lymph node resections (p. 54). Assessment of the patient with particular reference to groin dissection is as follows:

Hypotensive anaesthesia is available for this operation, and in order to be thoroughly safe careful assessment of the patient's cardiovascular state must be made. Two units of blood may be required for transfusion. The anaesthetic used in most of these patients has been an epidural block together with a light general anaesthetic.

The patient lies supine with a slight head downwards tilt. The drapes are placed in such a way that both legs can be moved if necessary during the operation without disturbing the sterility of the field. An in-dwelling Foley catheter is inserted with a drainage bag connected to it. The perineum and genitalia are covered with a dry abdominal pack. The leg on the affected side is placed so that the sole of the foot lies against the medial aspect of the opposite knee or mid calf.

Operation

The line of spread is marked from the primary tumour towards the inguinal lymph nodes or main lymphatic vessels in the thigh. In many cases, this is not difficult to do while in others, e.g. a lesion on the lateral aspect of the calf, the exact line of spread is indeterminate, and a compromise consists of marking one of the two most direct routes from the primary tumour to the major lymphatics in the thigh. The line of spread for lesions situated on the thigh is directly to a point approximately 3 cm below the inguinal ligament, i.e. roughly the centre of the inguinal lymph nodes. The line of spread is taken to be that line which most closely approximates the venous drainage from the area of the tumour to these sites. The incisions are marked out by identifying the anterior superior iliac spine laterally and the pubic tubercle medially and drawing in the line of the inguinal ligament. The area of skin and subcutaneous tissues containing the major thigh lymph trunks is then marked out along the line of the saphenous vein to a point about 5 cm above the knee.

The abdominal incision begins above the inguinal ligament and extends laterally about 2 cm above and parallel to the iliac crest, for about 6 cm. This incision is then carried above the inguinal ligament to the pubic tubercle. Small extensions of this incision are made downwards into the thigh along the predetermined marks. It is unnecessary to extend the incisions down into the leg until the intra-abdominal portion of the operation has been completed. The incision on the abdominal wall above the iliac crest is made with the knife held at right angles to the skin (an access incision). The remainder of the incisions which surround the possible tumour-bearing tissue are made with the knife held aslant the skin at an angle of 45 degrees to undercut away from the site of the nodes and lymphatics ('cancer ablative incisions').

The dissection commences by clearing the fat and fascia from the external oblique aponeurosis and muscle. The superficial epigastric, the external pudendal and superficial circumflex vessels are identified as they cross the wound and are ligated. Once the surface of the external oblique aponeurosis is exposed, the surgeon follows this structure until it has been cleared to the level of the iliac crest laterally and the whole length of the inguinal ligament medially. The risk of damage to the femoral vessels is minimised if the inguinal ligament is first identified at the medial end, close to the pubic tubercle near to the femoral canal. If in error the surgeon cuts too deeply at the medial end close to the incision, the only bleeding encountered is from a cluster of small vessels entering the surface of the pectineus muscle. As the dissection proceeds laterally along the inguinal ligament, the blue colour of the femoral vein is recognised more easily than the femoral artery. The femoral nerve lying behind the fascia iliaca is not visualised at this stage. A Kocher retractor is inserted beneath the inguinal ligament lateral to the femoral artery and the ligament is retracted upwards. Two pairs of vessels are identified and ligated: (1) The deep circumflex iliac artery and vein pass laterally, and when the ligament is displaced upwards, they may be lower than anticipated; accidental division can cause irritating haemorrhage. (2) The inferior epigastric artery and vein on the deep aspect of the muscles are isolated by passing a finger behind the muscles from lateral to medial across the front of the external iliac vessels. In order to gain access to the external and internal iliac region the abdominal muscles and the inguinal ligament are divided at a point starting just medial to the anterior superior iliac spine and extending through the ligament and the abdominal muscles parallel to and 1 cm above the iliac crest. When this is complete, the peritoneum can be elevated from the iliac fossa. Dever retractors hold the peritoneum off the iliac fossa. As the retractors are inserted, note the testicular vessels passing upwards and the vas deferens passing medially; these structures are preserved. The operability can now be assessed by the size and extent of the intra-abdominal lymphatic spread.

Dissection of the lymph nodes commences laterally and the fat and fascia from the iliac fossa are reflected towards the main vessels. The lateral cutaneous nerve of the thigh will be seen close to anterior superior iliac spine. The femoral branch of the genitofemoral nerve is identified and divided; it lies anterior to the femoral nerve. The femoral nerve should be identified early in this dissection, although it lies behind the plan of the dissection, posterior to the fascia iliaca. The nerve has a somewhat variable position: it may be 2 cm lateral to the femoral artery and partly concealed in a fold of the iliopsoas muscle, or it may be almost behind the femoral artery. If there is any difficulty in finding the femoral nerve, it is best to find the branch entering the deep aspect of the sartorius muscle about 4 to 6 cm below the line of the inguinal ligament and follow it upwards to the main trunk. The common error in identifying the femoral nerve is to look for it too far laterally. Once the nerve has been found, the dissection of the lateral aspect of the vessels is completed safely. The adventitia of the iliac artery is then freed together with the lymph trunks and nodes on all aspects of the vessel.

Similar dissection is then executed around the external iliac vein. Note these points during the dissection:

1. Apart from the two branches already mentioned, there are usually no branches encountered of the external iliac artery, but it may be difficult to accurately estimate the level

of the dissection when the inguinal ligament and abdominal muscles are retracted. The external iliac artery may be lifted with a Kocher retractor to facilitate the dissection on its posterior and medial aspects.

2. The external iliac vein is tethered at the upper end by the commencement of the internal iliac vein.

3. The obturator vein frequently arises from the medial side of the external iliac vein and crosses the superior ramus of the pubis to reach the obturator foramen. It is easy to damage this vein if its path lies further forwards than usual. The vein should be identified and divided between ligatures before clearing the medial aspect of the external iliac vein.

4. The lymph vessels lie very close to the main blood vessels and unless the outer layers of the adventitia are removed, major lymph trunks may be divided. There are frequently small lymph nodes lying between or behind the major blood vessels; it is therefore important to strip these of their adventitia on all surfaces.

5. In the upper part of the dissection the ureter will be seen.

6. To reach the nodes within the true pelvis, the position of the retractors must be altered; two broad Dever retractors are used, one holds the peritoneum medially and the second holds it upwards. It is difficult to make this part of the dissection in continuity. First, start as far posteriorly as possible and separate the fat, fascia and contained lymph nodes from the medial pelvic wall by *blunt* dissection. While doing this, note the following:

a. The ureter should be held wide of the operative field.

b. There is frequently a lymph node close to the obturator nerve near the obturator foramen. This node may cause some confusion because it is often long and thin and resembles a tubular structure, but by dissecting around it its true nature can be determined.

c. When the dissection is proceeding, the obturator nerve will be seen to be clear of the pelvic wall and free of surrounding tissue.

d. There may be some bleeding from the superior vesical vessels; this is usually venous and is easily controlled with a pack inserted into the pelvis while the remainder of the operation is completed. The retractors are removed and the tissues from the region reflected into the thigh.

The skin incisions are now continued down the thigh, the skin being undercut as before. As the thigh is abducted and rotated, the saphenous vein lies more medially than may be expected so that the lower central point where the incisions meet is opposite the line of the sartorius muscle, which is posterior to the medial femoral condyle and about 6 to 8 cm proximal to it.

Dissection of the groin proper begins on the lateral aspect. The deep fascia over the insertion of the sartorius is divided downwards along the lateral border of the muscle and the small branches of the lateral circumflex artery and vein are sealed with diathermy or ligated and divided. The deep fascia of the thigh separates easily from the sartorius. The nerve to the sartorius has been referred to, and further down the intermediate and medial cutaneous nerve of the thigh may pierce the muscle near its medial edge. The nerve to the vastus medialis may be seen lying behind the cutaneous nerves if the subsartorial canal is opened; this nerve should be preserved. However, the medial and intermediate cutaneous nerves will restrict adequate clearance of the upper part of the thigh and there is little morbidity from their loss; they are divided close to their origin. Small laterally running branches of the femoral artery will be seen passing between the divisions of the femoral nerve; these are divided at their origin from the femoral artery and, provided none is disturbed in the subsartorius canal, the blood supply to the upper part of the sartorius will be satisfactory. When dissection of the lateral aspect of the thigh is almost complete the anterior aspect of the femoral artery is systematically cleared from above downwards. A series of small arteries arising from the front of the femoral artery will be encountered and ligated flush with the main vessel, the lateral femoral circumflex at its origin (if this has not been seen already), the superficial epigastric, and on the medial side the external pudendal artery. These vessels have all been seen and ligated in the edges of the wound early in the operation. Distal to these vessels are two or three small unnamed arteries that arise from the front of the femoral artery and pass into the region of the lymph nodes in the femoral triangle. The nerve to the pectineus passes behind the femoral artery, and when dissecting in this region the nerve should be preserved. Just below this level the large profunda femoris artery will be seen to be passing slightly lateral and posterior to the main vessels.

Attention is now directed to the medial side of the operative field. The medial limit of the dissection is marked out at the upper end by the pubic tubercle and distal to this by the anterior border of the gracilis muscle. The superior ramus of the pubis is cleared of all tissues down to the periosteum. During this dissection, note the femoral vein is tethered on its posterior aspect by the branches from the pectineus and adductor muscles. The vein is easily compressed, and unless care is taken to avoid injury it is a simple matter to slit its medial wall. After the medial aspect of the femoral vein has been cleared for about 4 cm the surgeon dissects the front of the vein. As he proceeds downwards, clearing the adventitia from the femoral vein, the vein appears to thicken. This thickening heralds the entrance of the saphenous vein. The saphenous vein is doubly ligated proximally, clamped distally, and divided beyond both ligatures. The remainder of the operation is a simple matter of removing all the fat and fascia from the front of the femoral triangle. During the lower part of the dissection, the cutaneous division of the obturator nerve will be seen emerging between the gracilis and the medial border of adductor longus. When the dissection is complete all the muscles and the femoral vessels should be bare of all connective tissue. Haemostasis is checked, particularly in the pelvis, and closure begins.

The abdominal muscles are closed downwards using interrupted 2/0 Supramid stitches. Points to observe in closure are: Do not repair the anatomy of the region in an attempt to return it to normal. The abdominal wall will be less tense if the repair slightly reduces the length of the path taken by the abdominal muscles and inguinal ligament from the pubic tubercle laterally. The medial end of the inguinal ligament is closed to the superior ramus of the pubis and the pectineus muscle. The ligament is then lightly closed around the femoral artery and vein. It is important when the ligament is being closed on the fascia iliaca to be sure that no part of a stitch catches the femoral nerve. The nerve is avoided by passing a finger of the left hand between the nerve and the fascia with the pulp of the finger lying on the nerve. The passage of the needle through the fascia can easily be directed without any risk of damage to the nerve. The remaining parts of the incision lateral to this point are closed in the same way and care must be taken to avoid the lateral cutaneous nerve of the thigh at the lateral end of the inguinal ligament. The sartorius muscle is now transposed across the front of the femoral vessels (Baronofsky, 1948). This is done by dividing the muscle at its origin. In the upper end of the sartorius there is an intramuscular tendon. This is grasped and the muscle rotated on its long axis so that the lateral edge of the sartorius comes to lie over the medial aspect of the femoral vein. While the assistant holds the muscle in the correct position, any restraining bands of fibrous tissue on the deep surface of the muscle are divided. A few vessels will be seen entering the muscle; these should be preserved. Using a continuous 3/0 atraumatic chromic catgut stitch which commences at the former medial border of the sartorius, this muscle is attached successively to the iliopsoas, the external oblique aponeurosis just above the inguinal ligament, the pectineus and finally the adductor longus. The femoral vessels have now been completely covered with healthy muscle.

Before the skin is closed, the position of the leg must be returned to the resting position. If this is not done, the suture closing the skin to the underlying muscle may tear out when the position of the leg is altered and the dressing applied. The incision in the lower part of the thigh can be closed by direct apposition. The skin of the abdominal wall is closed with interrupted 3/0 black silk stitches as far medially as the anterior superior iliac spine. There remains the long triangular gap in the upper thigh. This space is narrowed by closing the skin to the underlying muscle with a continuous 2/0 atraumatic Dexon stitch which apposes the skin on to the underlying muscle.

A split skin graft is taken from the opposite thigh and held in place over the raw area by interrupted 3/0 black silk stitches. Modest pressure is applied to the graft by a 1-inch thick plastic foam sheet cut to the shape of the defect. No drainage is used.

The dressings are applied with the thigh flexed about 20 degrees. the foot and calf are swathed in cottonwool and, using a 6-inch crêpe bandage, the whole limb from the base of the knee is firmly supported up to the fold of the groin. Firm pressure on the graft is maintained by Elastoplast (3 inch) applied around the thigh and up over the abdomen.

Postoperative management

1. The patient is given 500 000 units of penicillin 6-hourly for three days.

2. The leg on the affected side is supported on a pillow, with a cradle protecting the foot from the weight of the bedclothes.

3. The foot of the bed is raised on 6-inch blocks.

4. The physiotherapist attends the patient at least daily to instruct him in breathing exercises and movement of the toes and ankle. The latter is not moved if the skin graft has been applied to the calf.

5. Unless there is evidence of wound infection or of profuse discharge, and both are unlikely, the dressings are not touched for six days.

6. The patient is sat out of bed in three days and he commences walking in a frame after six days.

7. As soon as possible after the patient is mobile, he is given a shower and washed with antiseptic soap, the donor site being protected from water by means of a plastic cover which is applied over the bandage. The operation site is allowed to get wet and is cleaned with Tincture of Metaphen after the area has been dried. Occasionally the junction between the graft and the skin edge develops excessive granulation tissue which can be reduced with powdered copper sulphate application to the area.

8. The average duration of hospitalisation is $2\frac{1}{2}$ weeks after operation.

9. If minor wound attention is needed after this period, it is carried out either by a home visiting nurse or preferably by a near relative.

10. The patient is instructed to wear a full-length elastic stocking from the moment he gets out of bed. He removes the stocking only when he takes his evening shower or bath. It is important to stress this because if the patient leaves the stocking off and the leg unsupported for a prolonged period, it may result in swelling which can be difficult to reduce. Six months after operation if the lymphoedema is slight, the patient commences to leave the stocking off. The way this is done is important if oedema is to be kept to a minimum. The patient is asked to remove the stocking first at the end of the day, say about the time of the evening meal. If, when he has done this for three consecutive days, the leg has not swollen by the time he goes to bed each night, he is asked to remove the stocking a couple of hours earlier for another three days. The process is repeated as he gradually lengthens the period when he is free of the stocking, commencing in the evening until he can go a full day without its support. However, the patient is warned not to undertake any prolonged and unaccustomed standing, e.g. serving in a shop, when he has only recently discarded the stocking. The patient is also warned that in very hot weather the leg may become swollen and he may need the stocking support at such times.

Comments

1. The usual time for one of these operations is three hours. The blood loss from swab weight has varied from 187 to 800 ml, the average being approximately 400 ml. The key

factor in this low blood loss is a hypotensive anaesthetic and the use of the diathermy mentioned in Chapter 3. During most of the dissecting part of the operation, i.e. the first half, the systolic blood pressure should vary between 70 to 80 mmHg. The amount of bleeding increases substantially if the systolic blood pressure passes 90 to 199 mmHg.

2. Insertion of the catheter has been found useful partly because after epidural anaesthesia, patients tend to have urinary retention for two to three days and partly because the retained catheter keeps the dressings cleaner during the first few days.

3. Lymphoedema is the one troublesome complication of radical inguinal lymph node resection, and in recent years I have tried several techniques in an effort to reduce this without interfering with the principles of the operation in relation to cancer. It would be premature to claim these efforts have been successful, although the impression is lymphoedema is less of a problem now than formerly. The techniques tried have been to dissect out two or three major lymphatics and to implant them into a vein or muscle. This proved very time-consuming after an already lengthy operation. An easier method and one which appears equally as effective is to demonstrate the position of some major lymphatics, wide of the line of spread, and to cut a small trough in the muscles which lie close to these vessels. The subcutaneous tissues are then invaginated into this raw muscle with a continuous plain catgut suture (2/0), which passes first along one lip of the trough and the deep fascia then along the other surface and the subcutaneous tissues close to the skin. In this way the lymphatics 'bleed' directly into the muscle bellies and it is hoped this will allow easy absorption of the lymph.

Complications

The complications of ilio-inguinal lymphadenectomy can be divided into four groups: immediate, delayed, local in the affected leg and general complications which apply to all surgery.

IMMEDIATE—WOUND BREAKDOWN

It used to be taught, or if not taught implied, that the skin of the groin had some mildly malevolent characteristics because it 'healed badly', and indeed any adequate dissection of the groin is likely to be followed by a sloughing of the skin. Having observed this on several occasions in patients seen many years ago, I evolved a technique of primary split skin grafting to groin operations (Milton, 1963) after the following observations had been made:

1. The skin of the front of the thigh which sloughs after groin dissection is nearly always below the line of the inguinal ligament and, as a rule, will extend for a distance of up to 8 to 12 cm down the leg. The skin on either side of the wound may slough.

2. The blood supply to the skin of the front of the thigh may be seen to come from three to five small branches arising from the femoral artery. These may either arise separately from the sides or front of the femoral artery, or one or more of them may have a common origin before they divide. Beneath the cribriform fascia, three of these arteries are dignified with names, the superficial external pudendal, the superficial epigastric and the superficial circumflex iliac artery. In addition to these named arteries, there are one or two unnamed vessels arising from the anterior surface of the femoral artery down to the point where the artery lies beneath the sartorius muscle, and it is at this point that a major branch arises from the superficial femoral artery and descends in the subcutaneous tissues near the saphenous vein, i.e. the descending genicular artery. Any adequate groin dissection must remove all branches down to but not including the descending genicular artery, and when this is done, the devascularisation of the skin of the thigh is inevitable. The devascularisation, however, is largely in the skin as the slough does not extend deeply into the subcutaneous fat.

ACCIDENTAL BURN

If the lateral cutaneous nerve of the thigh has been divided, the patient must be warned that he has an anaesthetic area on the outer thigh and he must be careful not to apply radiant heat to any part of the wound. There have been two occasions when the patient on discharge home felt that the slight weeping at the edges of the skin graft could be dried with a warm lamp and in both cases caused an unpleasant but painless burn which took a long time to heal.

LYMPHOEDEMA

This has been mentioned in this chapter together with methods of controlling it. However, several additional points need to be made in relation to this important sequalae of the operation.

1. The type of person who has the most severe leg swelling appears to be the short 'dumpy' woman, whereas tall and thin people are usually not severely affected. The reason for this difference is not apparent.

2. The lymphoedema certainly worsens in very hot weather and after prolonged standing.

3. A swollen leg will not affect a patient's ability to play athletic sports; indeed, activities such as tennis and golf appear to maintain a supple leg.

4. The swelling may be made worse if the patient develops recurrent bouts of streptococcal lymphangitis in the leg. The site of entry of the organisms is usually invisible, but minor abrasions on either the proximal or distal parts of the limb may enable the streptococci to enter.

5. Lymphangitis in the leg, as in the arm, tends to be recurrent unless penicillin (oral) is continued for two months after all clinical evidence of it has resolved.

6. A grossly oedematous leg can be considerably reduced in size by admitting the patient to hospital and nursing him with the leg elevated and compressed in an inflated air splint. The manner of applying the splint is to attach a $2\frac{1}{2}$-foot (75 cm) rubber tube to the inflating valve and the patient is asked to blow up the splint after it has been placed on the leg, in the same way as blowing up a balloon. The reason for this is that the amount of pressure the patient can generate is not enough to damage the circulation in the skin but it is enough to apply adequate pressure to reduce the swelling. The patient is also taught to measure the circumference of the limb at the calf and to keep a chart of its size. Once the limb has been shrunk in this way, the patient wears one or even two elastic stockings (one over the other) whenever he is up and about.

7. Operations for lymphoedema once it has become established are disappointing.

8. The use of elastic stockings is important if the swelling tends to become excessive. The stockings, to be effective, must fit well and be firm. The patient should always have a pair so that when one is being washed he has a clean one to apply. He should also devise a support which prevents the stocking from rolling down (especially in the thigh) when it tends to act as a tourniquet. The most satisfactory support is a 'girdle' around the waist with suspender straps hanging down at three or four points around the thigh.

GRAFT FAILURE AND WOUND INFECTION

These should both be minor problems which are handled in the usual way.

LATE LOCAL EFFECTS

Late local effects of lymphadenectomy have already been covered under the heading of 'Lymphoedema'.

GENERAL EFFECTS

The most worrying is pulmonary embolism but although so much of this dissection is in the region of the large veins, and immobility of the leg is a feature of the postoperative management, I have not had one case of fatal embolism; minor embolic episodes which can be easily diagnosed and require treatment occur about once in every 15 to 20 patients.

INGUINAL LYMPH NODE BIOPSY AND LYMPH FISTULA

There are occasions when a few of the inguinal lymph nodes are excised, e.g. supply tumour for immunotherapy or to exclude neoplastic involvement of palpable nodes. The technique of the operation is simple and does not require elaboration here, but I have seen several cases of troublesome lymph fistulae developing from the wound in such procedures.

The management of these patients is to immobilise the leg for two weeks between sand bags with the patient in bed. This may be adequate to allow the wound to heal while the lymph flow is minimal. If this fails, one of two methods will be successful.

1. Inject Patent Blue V 'upstream' from the fistula before operation and when the blue dye emerges from the fistula explore the wound and ligate the lymph vessels with fine black silk.

2. If this technique is unsuccessful a narrow (3 mm) Haemovac drainage tube is inserted into the wound through a separate stab wound laterally in the thigh. The skin of the biopsy wound is carefully closed. The drainage tube is attached to a portable Haemovac spring suction. The patient is taught to empty and recharge the sucker and after a couple of days he goes home with instructions to empty the sucker three times a day. At first the lymph drainage continues unabated but after about a week to 10 days, it lessens and usually stops completely in three weeks. The tube is not removed for three to four more days.

RECURRENT MELANOMA IN THE THIGH REGION AFTER STANDARD INGUINAL LYMPHADENECTOMY

If melanoma recurs in the region of a standard inguinal node dissection it usually does so in one of three places:

1. In the scar of the operation.

2. Distal to the scar in line with the major lymphatics in the thigh close to one side of the scar.

3. In the external iliac nodes just above the inguinal ligament or in the obturator lymph nodes. I have seen two cases in whom the external iliac nodes were the seat of metastasis and who had no deposits of melanoma in the inguinal nodes. However, these 'skip' metastases are rare.

Results

The survival figures for ilio-inguinal lymph node dissection are given at the conclusion of Chapter 7 (p. 75). Local recurrence of disease within or close to the field of the operation is less than 5 per cent.

REFERENCES

Baronofsky, I. D. (1948) Technique of inguinal node dissection. *Surgery*, **24**, 555.
Milton, G. W. (1963) Some methods used in the management of metastatic malignant melanoma. *Australian Journal of Dermatology*, **7**, 15.

7. Melanoma of the Head and Neck

RADICAL DISSECTION OF CERVICAL LYMPH NODES

Treatment of melanoma on the head and neck is affected by factors similar to those which determine the treatment at other sites (p. 43).

1. *The type of melanoma*

a. Hutchinson's melanotic freckle becomes increasingly common on the head and neck in older people. Unlike other forms of melanoma it has little tendency to spread, hence lymph node resection is rarely necessary. HMF is usually a radiosensitive tumour, and the primary lesion can be satisfactorily treated with X-irradiation. If surgical excision is undertaken, it is unnecessary to excise wide areas of tissue but only remove the tumour and 3 to 5 mm of normal skin around the pigmented border. Occasionally in these patients a flat pigmented patch or freckle develops at the edge of the skin graft and extends very slowly across the graft and into the adjacent skin. The 'patch' often remains flat for long periods, and while it does so, no treatment is necessary. I have observed four such recurrent HMFs for up to five years in elderly patients and none came to surgery.

b. Nodular melanoma on the head and neck can be dangerous and the factors which affect treatment are:

    i. The age, general condition and wishes of the patient.
    ii. The site of the lesion and probable direction of lymph flow.
    iii. The extent of the tumour including the depth of penetration of the primary lesion and the evidence, if any, of metastasis.

The manner in which general factors influence the selection of treatment has been discussed on pages 43 and 54.

2. *The site of the melanoma*

The site of the primary lesion may indicate the site of expected lymph node metastases. The following observations are of a general nature but are difficult to place in numerical sequence. Melanoma in the scalp within an area roughly limited by the frontal eminences anteriorly and an equivalent site posteriorly may spread to either side of the upper deep cervical chain or parotid nodes. However, tumours in the scalp tend to recur near the original lesion and often no directional pattern can be demonstrated. Scalp melanoma also may metastasise by the bloodstream at an early stage. Lesions on the ear spread to the deep cervical nodes on the same side and also recur in the sulcus between the ear and the mastoid region. Melanoma on the forehead within about 3 cm of the mid-line may spread to either side (parotid lymph nodes), while those on the temple region involve the ipsilateral superficial parotid lymph nodes. Primary tumours in the conjunctiva, eyelids or the cheek involve the submandibular lymph nodes near the facial artery. Cross-over spread from lesions on the face is probably rare; I have seen it once. Melanoma on the neck spread to adjacent lymph nodes on the same side. The lower cervical (supraclavicular) nodes also draw lymph from the shoulder region (i.e. over the trapezius, above the spine of the scapula) on the same side.

3. *Depth of penetration*

The depth of penetration also influences the type of surgery recommended. If the lesion penetrates deeply into the reticular dermis or beyond and the draining nodes can be predicted, then I advise resection and if possible incontinuity. This applies especially in men where the prognosis is worse than for women. Bilateral radical cervical lymphadenectomy has never been recommended because the only lesions where this might be indicated would be the central scalp or forehead.

Melanoma in both these sites has some predeliction for blood spread. (Note: When these cases are broken down into groups of tumours affecting limited areas, e.g. central forehead, there are not enough personal cases to record meaningful figures.) Prophylactic lymph node resection is therefore recommended on the basis of the criteria given in the last paragraph, but palpable lymph nodes felt for the first time at follow-up should certainly be resected if the patient's general condition warrants it.

Radical dissection of cervical lymph nodes

The preoperative assessment and management follows the same pattern as that outlined for both axillary and inguinal lymphadenectomy (p. 54).

The operation follows the standard technique described in many textbooks, so I will concentrate on those points which are especially relevant to melanoma of the head and neck.

Melanoma of the head and neck appears to have a singular tendency to recur locally in the site of the cervical lymph node dissection, when compared to thorough dissections of the axilla or groin. Consequently, protection against seeding into the wound is important. Although cercival recurrence is more likely if the lymph nodes contain metastatic tumour, it can occur even when the excised nodes are negative. Local recurrence is in the tissue planes of the neck deep to the platysma and is not usually associated with the edge of the scar but tends to lie under the flaps.

The incisions used in this operation are those described in standard works but may be adapted to include the site of the primary lesion, if this is feasible. The best cosmetic result is obtained from two parallel incisions 4 to 6 cm apart lying in the skin creases of the neck. Access to the supraclavicular region is enhanced by extending the posterior end of the lower incision downwards to the region of the acromioclavicular joint, while the submental region can be thoroughly displayed by a vertical extension to the anterior end of the upper incision.

The cervical branch of the facial nerve should be preserved when it does not lie in the line of spread of the tumour. Identification of the nerve can be troublesome. The nerve may lie lower in the neck than expected and as the upper flap is raised it is easily damaged. The course of the nerve can be plotted by electrical stimulation of the region, and this is best done before the incision has been made. The easiest way to demonstrate the site of the nerve is to place one electrode of a stimulator well down the neck and apply a second electrode at various points, working from below upwards while watching the angle of the mouth. Each stimulus will produce a contraction of the platysma muscle between the electrodes by direct stimulation but a definite twitch of the angle of the mouth indicates a transmitted impulse along the cervical branch of the facial nerve. If this routine is followed in three to four places the course of the nerve can be drawn on the skin. Demonstration of the nerve beneath the platysma can be facilitated by distending the tissue plane just deep to the muscle with POR 9 (Sandoz) 1 : 40 ml saline. It is important not to use local anaesthetic with adrenalin because this will prevent any additional electrical stimulation being used to demonstrate the nerve.

The thoracic duct is easily damaged during dissection in the lower medial part of the operation. If the patient has been fasted, injury to the duct will be followed by a small amount of watery fluid accumulating in the angle between the internal jugular and subclavian veins. If there is any doubt concerning trauma to the thoracic duct, it is my practice to demonstrate and ligate it with fine black silk. The lymph from the ligated thoracic duct 'finds its way back to the bloodstream by collaterals or other lymphatico-venus communication' (Yoffey and Courtice, 1970).

Injury to the thoracic duct not recognised at operation may result in a lymph fistula from the medial end of the lower wound; if the fistula does not heal spontaneously within a few days, the patient is fasted for 24 hours allowing him enough water by mouth to quench his thirst. He is then maintained on a diet consisting largely of carbohydrates and fruit for a week.

The thoracic duct in the neck is closely associated with one or two small lymph nodes which may be stained black with carbon filtered from the pulmonary lymph. Macroscopically the dark nodes appear to be involved with melanoma, but a frozen section examination will demonstrate the presence of carbon and the absence of tumour cells.

Melanoma on the top of the shoulder or above the spine of the scapula can be resected incontinuity with the supraclavicular lymph nodes, i.e. the lower third to a half of a radical neck dissection. The few points of technique which are different from the standard neck dissection are as follows:

1. The clavicular head of the sternomastoid is divided about 1 cm above and parallel to the clavicle, care being taken to avoid injury to the small veins behind the muscle. The divided part of the muscle is held towards the opposite side while the lower end of the internal jugular vein is identified and preserved.

2. The dissection then proceeds backwards across the floor of the neck after dividing the transverse cervical artery and vein between ligatures.

3. The anterior fibres of the trapezius muscle are divided above and parallel to the clavicle for about 2 cm and the anterior border of the muscle is cleared of attachment to the cervical fascia and folded backwards. The point of entry of the spinal accessory (XI) nerve into the muscle is identified and the nerve dissected free of vessels surrounding it.

4. The posterior part of the dissection is now completed and the trapezius muscle reattached.

Complications of the operation

WOUND BREAKDOWN

This is a rare complication because the blood supply to the skin of the neck and face is profuse. In one patient a badly constructed flap necrosed and required excision and repair. In a small number of patients (not recorded) the posterior end of the lower incision opened up when the patient turned his head forcibly towards the opposite side. The posterior 3 to 4 cm of the lower wound was subjected to strain and this caused the wound edges to separate. This complication has been avoided by using slightly stronger skin sutures in the posterior end of the lower incision (i.e. 3/0 black silk as opposed to 5/0 black silk elsewhere), and leaving these sutures in place for 10 days (the remaining sutures are removed in 5 days).

GENERAL COMPLICATIONS

These are rare following neck dissection because the patient is allowed out of bed on the first or second postoperative day and has few restrictions to normal activity from that time onwards (see Results, p. 75).

MORBIDITY

The morbidity of radical dissection of cervical lymph nodes is mentioned in most textbooks of operative surgery and I will mention them briefly here:

1. The lower part of the face is often slightly oedematous for a few days after operation. The oedema is not serious because it subsides rapidly.

2. The shoulder on the affected side droops because of the division of the accessory nerve and consequent paralysis of the trapezius muscle. The weakness of the trapezius appears to cause no serious symptoms because no patient has complained of an inability to work or to play sport because of it.

3. The scars and the hollow in the neck on the affected side may cause the patient transient anxiety, but minor modification of dress is all that is necessary to conceal them. The scar of the skin graft on the face of women is best concealed with cosmetics.

Results

Figures 7.1, 7.2 and 7.3 show the survival figures of all lymph node dissections done at the clinic. The average survival for all cases of lymph node dissection is better than 60 per cent. The site of the primary tumour influences the outcome, the leg and arm being the most favourable site while the trunk and the head and neck are the most dangerous. These findings agree with most of the reported figures quoted elsewhere in this book. The explanation for the difference in survival for melanoma at different sites is not clear, e.g. it does not appear to be directly related to the size of the lesion. In all figures only nodular melanoma was considered. Hutchinson's melanotic freckle was excluded and superficial lesions did not undergo lymph node dissections.

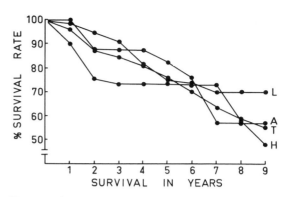

Fig. 7.2 Shows the survival figures of men following lymph node dissection and excision of primary melanoma. The site of the primary lesion is indicated: L = Leg, A = arm, T = trunk, H = head or neck.

Note: The leg is the most favourable site while the head and neck is the most dangerous.

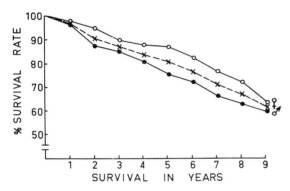

Fig. 7.1 Shows the survival figures (actuarial calculation) for all lymph node dissections carried out at the clinic. It includes all patients traced who died of melanoma, but excludes from all calculations patients lost to follow-up or who died of causes other than melanoma. The overall survival figure is better for women than for men, although it is not statistically significant at nine years.

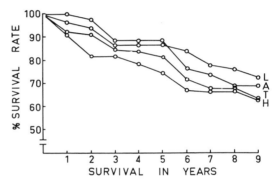

Fig. 7.3 Shows the survival of women following lymph node dissection and excision of the primary melanoma. The letters indicating the site of the primary lesion are as in Figure 7.2. Once more the leg is the most favourable site, while the trunk and head and neck the most dangerous.

REFERENCES

Yoffey, J. M. & Courtice, F. C. (1970) *Lymphatics, Lymph and the Lymphomyeloid Complex*, p. 383. London: Academic Press.

8. Clinical Features of Metastases

Figure 8.1 shows the site and time of recurrent malignant melanoma in 100 cases referred with recurrent disease (Milton, 1963). In about 75 per cent of the patients in whom the disease recurs, the first recurrence is at the site of the primary, in the intransit area or in the drainage

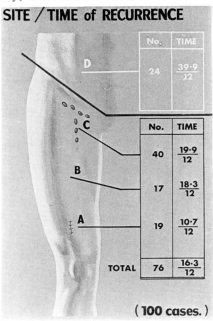

SITE / TIME of RECURRENCE

	No.	TIME
D	24	$\frac{39 \cdot 9}{12}$

	No.	TIME
	40	$\frac{19 \cdot 9}{12}$
	17	$\frac{18 \cdot 3}{12}$
	19	$\frac{10 \cdot 7}{12}$
TOTAL	76	$\frac{16 \cdot 3}{12}$

(**100 cases.**)

Fig. 8.1   Shows the site and time of the first detected recurrence of melanoma in 100 patients with metastatic disease. To simplify the diagram, it has been drawn as if the primary tumours were all on the thigh. Actually, they were widely distributed. A represents the site of the primary lesion; B the line of spread—i.e. intransit deposits; C the first draining lymph nodes; D implies a first recurrence beyond the lymphatic drainage area—i.e. a central recurrence such as in the liver, lungs, brain or disseminated in subcutaneous tissues. The time indicates the average number of months from the first definitive treatment to diagnosis of the metastasis.

lymph nodes (40 per cent). In the remaining quarter of patients, the first sign of recurrence is detected at some central point, such as the lungs or liver or distant subcutaneous sites. On average, the nearer the recurrence to the site of the primary lesion the sooner it is diagnosed. At first sight these figures might suggest that the spread of melanoma was a sequential advance from one position to the next, but this is not established by these findings.

The factors which determine the development of metastases are not well understood. Some anatomical features of the primary lesion affecting the chance of any form of dissemination appear fairly straightforward, e.g. usually the deeper it penetrates below the epidermal basement membrane, the more dangerous it is (p. 15) (Clark et al., 1969; McLeod et al., 1971). The explanation of the type of metastases and the time they take to develop remains a matter for speculation. In some cases a long latent interval from the primary excision to the diagnosis of metastasis could be explained on the growth rate of the tumour, for example a few melanocytes in the liver may need years to grow large enough to cause a detectable mass, while the same number of cells seeded in a peripheral lymph node become palpable much sooner. Unfortunately, this is not likely to be the correct answer in every instance. Another mystery is why some lesions metastasise in a selective way, e.g. an enlarged liver with no other sign of disease, or multiple subcutaneous and few visceral deposits.

One way to discuss these problems is to suggest that a kind of dialogue or 'language' develops between the tumour and the host. The 'language' must be subtle as it is presumably chemical and in part related to immune mechanisms. However, the receptors required to understand this language are still rudimentary. Before discussing the clinical attributes of spreading melanoma, I wish to place a few speculations about the characteristics of the participants of this dialogue.

The tumour. A clinically diagnosed cancer (e.g. melanoma) must have certain characteristics in relation to the host. The tumour must not set up any effective rejection response in the host, because if it did the small mass of tumour in early development would be destroyed by the host. The tumour mass need not be homogeneous functionally (even if it looks so histologically). As the tumour develops and mutants arise in it, any mutant cell which does not have the innate power of survival and the capacity to avoid triggering the host's defences would be destroyed. The growing tumour or metastasis must also be adaptable to changing or different environments or it will not survive. So a form of natural selection occurs in a developing tumour. The same form of natural selection will operate in every collection of tumour cells which lodge at a possible site for metastasis. If the local immune mechanisms detect some cells they may be destroyed; others without the same attributes survive. Just as the primary tumour is likely to be polyclonal, so are the metastases.

From the host's point of view, the more effective his defence mechanisms the better. But his defences are apparently not the same in all his tissues. So it comes about that selective survival of tumour cells is possible in one organ or tissue. In addition, the host's defences may be generally disturbed, e.g. by immune suppression.

Hence the 'dialogue' between host and tumour has the possibility of an immense number of variables. It is likely that these are not static and so a continually fluctuating struggle between two living systems evolves, governed by the rules of natural selection.

1. Subcutaneous and intracutaneous metastases

These most commonly present by the patient feeling a painless lump in or under the skin. If the metastasis is in the skin, it is usually discoloured.

Subcutaneous and intracutaneous metastases may be either blood or lymph borne. Those deposits occurring far away from the site of the primary tumour and not related to the draining lymph vessels are presumably blood borne. The so-called 'intransit' metastasis is likely to be in lymph vessels. The position of the metastasis in relation to the primary tumour is of some importance when discussing treatment. The first detectable metastasis on the trunk or a limb anatomically related to the primary tumour is nearly always close to the line of spread from the site of the primary to the draining lymph nodes. However, there are some exceptions:

a. If a node dissection has resulted in lymphoedema the secondaries in that limb may occur initially wide of the line of spread, even distal to the primary site.

b. When the metastases grow and become more profuse they spread out and become widely distributed in the limb.

c. One patient had cardiac failure and severe oedema of both legs and developed all his limb recurrences distal to the primary lesion.

Although the usual presentation of a subcutaneous deposit is a painless lump, there are two other less common methods of presentation. In some patients who have been given immunotherapy and, very rarely, in otherwise untreated patients, the subcutaneous nodule appears to be inflammatory (i.e. tender, hot and painful).

The second unusual method of presentation of a subcutaneous nodule is for the patient to develop a spontaneous bruise and a lump becomes palpable at the centre of this as it resolves. This sequence of events is not always associated with rapid and generalised disease although it usually is.

Melanomatous deposits in fat may occur in any site, but usually cause no symptoms unless a palpable lump is observed. However, the growing metastasis in a confined space may cause symptoms, e.g. diplopia or nerve root pain.

2. Lymph nodes

Characteristic clinical features of malignant melanoma in the lymph nodes differ from those of squamous cell carcinoma or adenocarcinomatous nodes. The features of melanoma-involved nodes are as follows. The node is often noticed first by the patient and it appears to have developed suddenly. After the patient first noticed it, the node usually does not appear to enlarge even over several weeks, and he will often comment that the lump seems to be getting smaller; repeated clinical examination confirms this. The node is usually not tender but may become so, particularly if the patient is worried about it. On clinical examination, the node tends to be firm, rather like a solitary node of Hodgkin's disease, not hard like those involved with other forms of cancer. The node is usually felt singly but there may be more than one demonstrable histologically. The node does not become attached to surrounding tissues even when it is large, hence it will nearly always feel mobile. Nodes of immense size pressing against the skin may

produce obvious discolouration. It is also important to notice at operation that occasionally adjacent lymph nodes will be black, because they have absorbed melanin from an isolated and massive metastasis. Left untouched, the patient usually does not survive long enough for the nodes to fungate through the skin. The condition of the primary tumour does not appear to determine the size of the nodes (Fig. 8.2). In fact, in occult primary melanoma the original tumour may have been completely destroyed while the nodal metastases develop rapidly.

The site of involved lymph nodes usually follows a predictable pattern early in the disease. The watersheds are roughly as follows. On the back above the waist, a lesion within the line marked by the lateral border of the erector spinae muscles may metastasise to either axilla. Lateral to this line it will nearly always spread first to the ipsilateral side. Above the spine of the scapula the first metastasis is to the root of the neck. Anteriorly presumably a similar watershed exists, although this has not been well shown in these cases. The cranio-

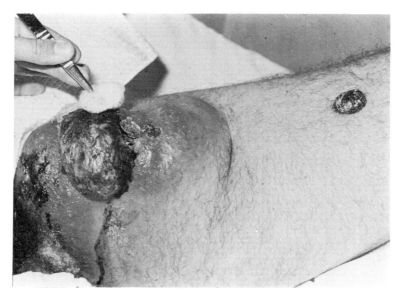

Fig. 8.2   Shows the great disparity which can occur between the primary tumour (Rt) and huge metastases in the draining lymph nodes. Nodal metastases of melanoma do not commonly fungate to this extent unless the area has been interfered with surgically.

caudal division between axillary and inguinal node drainage areas appears to be level with the umbilicus, those above spreading to the axilla. In the limbs the epitrochlea lymph node in the arm is frequently involved with lesions on the forearm, while the popliteal lymph nodes seem to be rarely involved. (This latter comment is not established and remains an impression.) In the head and neck, the watershed is usually the mid-line. The clavicle appears to form the borderline between the root of the neck and the axilla.

It seems to be rare for the first clinical involvement of lymph nodes to be detected beyond those nearest the tumour. One young man, with a small primary lesion on the lower lateral aspect of the thigh, presented with a palpable external iliac lymph node; the inguinal lymph nodes were not only impalpable but also negative for tumour after excision.

Involvement of lymph vessels may be affected by lymph stasis, when a form of melanoma *en cuirasse* may develop. However, most of these cases have had a lymphadenectomy and spread into the lymphatics has followed the operation.

3. Liver

Clinical features of liver involvement in melanoma develop in one of two ways. The fit patient may lose his appetite and the liver may remain impalpable for up to two months after this. The loss of appetite progresses into nausea and the nausea to vomiting and utter revulsion against food. The patient dies from a combination of starvation and liver failure. Secondly, with both occular and cutaneous melanoma, the liver involvement may be symptomless and the liver metastases are detected by routine palpation detecting an enlarged liver. The liver may reach considerable dimensions before the patient is aware of discomfort. He then feels a dragging sensation in the right side but does not show nausea or evidence of liver failure over a prolonged period. In one extraordinary case, a champion athlete in training for the Olympic Games had an obviously palpable liver due to secondary melanoma and at the same time his athletic performance measured by medical officers for the Olympic team was at the peak of physical fitness. Jaundice is not a common feature of liver involvement in the early stages. However, as the hepatic enlargement increases there is a tendency for jaundice to become apparent, but this may be masked by the development of a generalised grey-brown melanin pigmentation. Sometimes the liver metastases bleed and the patient feels a sudden pain under the right chest, but as a general rule hepatic metastases are not painful. In the later stages of liver metastases obstruction to the inferior vena cava may cause gross oedema of the genitals and legs.

4. Intestinal metastases

These usually involve the small intestine and the commonest presenting feature in these patients is recurrent bouts of central abdominal colic. In two patients the pain had been so persistent that they had been referred for psychiatric assessment. Anaemia due to repeated haemorrhage from mucosal metastasis is the second commonest presentation of bowel deposits. Two patients have presented with perforated bowel and symptoms of peritonitis and two others were sent to hospital with shock and features of peritonitis due to intraperitoneal haemorrhage from subserosal or omental metastasis. Secondary melanoma in the stomach causes expected symptoms of anaemia and loss of appetite, but they are less common than those in the small bowel.

5. Retroperitoneal metastases

These are painless except those involving the pancreas when the patient develops chronic, deep-seated abdominal pain which becomes more severe and penetrates through to the back in the course of two to three months.

6. Lung metastases

Symptoms produced by secondary deposits in the lung are determined by the position of the metastasis. If they abut the pleura the resultant effusion causes dyspnoea. If the metastases are in the bronchial mucosa the first symptom will be a dry unproductive cough. As the disease progresses, the patient coughs up black melanin as well as blood. Tumours involving the hilar lymph nodes cause progressive dyspnoea and cough. The commonest form of pulmonary metastasis is the 'cannon ball' deposit but diffuse infiltration of the lung has been seen.

7. Brain metastases

These present in a variety of guises which, of course, are common to other tumours. Firstly, there are those which present with clinical features of raised intracranial pressure, morning headache being the dominant symptom. As this progresses, failure of vision and disorientation follow. Secondly, symptoms of cerebral irritation, i.e. Jacksonian epilepsy (probably the commonest). Thirdly, symptoms due to cranial nerve (or nerve nuclei) involvement, such as diplopia or visual field defects. Visual defects may also be caused by retinal detachment resulting from metastasis. Diplopia can be caused by retro-ocular deposits displacing the globe forwards. Personality changes from frontal lobe metastasis no doubt could occur but has not been seen in the present series.

8. Spinal metastases

These are usually extradural and cause pain along a nerve root, which may be followed by the development of paraplegia. It is important to notice that the duration of pain before the paraplegia commences varies considerably; some patients have root pain for months and never develop paraplegia; however, if paraplegia develops, the onset is often very rapid. The initial symptom is either weakness of the legs and/or incontinence of urine. The time from the first symptom to complete paraplegia may be less than 48 hours. Spinal decompression once severe paraplegia has developed rarely produces much improvement.

9. Bony metastases

These generally follow the pattern of those of other tumours and there is frequently little correlation between the amount of bone destruction as seen on X-ray and the severity of the pain. The bone pain has all the characteristic features of secondary tumour in bone and the pain may be present for up to two months before there is X-ray evidence of bone involvement. Although the metastases may be sclerotic, the majority are osteoporotic.

10. Bladder and ureter metastases

These cause haematuria or filling defects seen on X-ray in the kidney or bladder.

RANDOM OBSERVATIONS

The observations which follow are difficult to neatly codify as required by science, and some of them are even anecdotal (if Dr Samuel Johnson were living as a scientific lexicographer he would surely have defined 'anecdotal' as 'a low word, not used by the erudite').

Figure 8.3 illustrates a feature of metastatic melanoma seen in most forms of metastases but especially those in subcutaneous tissues and lymph nodes. Melanoma does not permeate the tissues as other malignant tumours; it seeds into discrete, well-defined clusters which push the tissues aside rather than invade them.

The clinician is apt to think of expanding tumours as one mass of living growth, but attempts to culture cells from metastases show that 60 to 90 per cent of cells in them are dead (E. M. Stephenson, N. G. Stephenson, G. W. Milton, 1973, unpublished data). The cause of this cell morality could be simply a matter of blood supply, especially as most of the necrotic tissue tends to be in the middle of the tumour mass, but simple explanations have often been inaccurate. The question of host reaction in terms of clinical behaviour may be surmised but is hard to prove. The usual course for melanoma is to become disseminated while the primary disease remains small. However, there are occasional cases where massive local disease

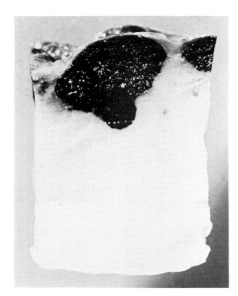

Fig. 8.3 Shows expanding melanoma metastasis in and beneath the skin. Note the well-defined edge and the absence of host reaction to the tumour. These attributes of spreading melanoma are occasionally useful in dealing with large secondary deposits, because they can be resected while similar deposits from squamous or adenocarcinoma would be irremovably fixed to surrounding tissues.

has not metastasised. Lewis (1972) has reviewed the literature as well as reporting his own findings, which suggest that this large local growth without spread is caused by a circulating antibody. It is of interest that this antibody is ineffective in destroying the primary tumour.

The host reaction to a melanoma or lack of it can be frequently seen at the edges of metastases. However, host reaction to the tumour may take other forms. Although it is not common for cutaneous metastasis to be surrounded by depigmentation, this does occur sometimes and takes one of two forms: a fairly large pale halo around some, but not all, deposits and a smaller more intense halo close to almost all secondaries. The latter is more frequent although it is usually more marked after effective treatment (e.g. with chemotherapy).

A more dramatic form of depigmentation has been seen in 13 patients who developed considerable vitiligo. Two of these patients had received chemotherapy but in the remainder the vitiligo developed spontaneously (Milton, McCarthy and Carlon, 1971). The main features of patients with vitiligo are:

1. The depigmentation develops at any site but is most easily seen on the hands and face, possibly because these areas are often tanned.

2. The position of the vitiligo may vary from time to time, one area becoming pigmented while another bleaches.

3. The vitiligo often develops while the patient has no clinical evidence of metastases, although most patients had had some evidence of dissemination, e.g. metastatic lymph nodes.

4. The melanoma had frequently followed an unusually prolonged course, but unfortunately 7 out of the 11 patients have died from recurrent melanoma which appeared less than 12 months after the vitiligo. Two patients remain alive.

5. No other cause for the vitiligo was apparent, i.e. no family history, no suggestion of other possibly auto-immune diseases such as thyrotoxicosis or diabetes mellitus.

It is reasonable to conclude that the appearance of vitiligo is not coincidental but is related to the immune 'dialogue' between host and tumour (Fig. 8.4).

There are even more obscure and rare forms of reaction between host and tumour. Small vessel arteritis causing Raynaud's phenomenon in the fingers and toes has been seen once—this patient also developed erythema multiforme six months later.

SPECIAL TESTS FOR SECONDARY MELANOMA

It would be of great benefit if it were possible to detect the secondary spread of melanoma by a test which was more sensitive and more reliable than a careful history and physical examination. The detection of latent metastases is difficult and, except for the chest X-ray, not reliable. The history and physical examination are typical in patients who develop subcutaneous nodules. Biopsy may be useful to prove the diagnosis but there is no point in doing this more than once. Lung metastases are well revealed on X-ray.

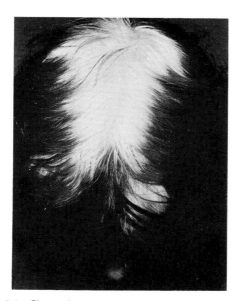

Fig. 8.4   Shows the crown of a 23-year-old woman who 12 months before had had a melanoma removed from her shoulder and a radical axillary dissection performed. The lower nodes in the axilla contained tumour. She remained well and apparently free of disease and then rapidly developed vitiligo. Four months after this she had the first symptoms of cerebral metastasis, from which she died. Note the sudden transition between normal and white hair, which presumably represents a change in the host/tumour or host/pigment relationship. Hair on the crown grows at between 0·45 and 0·5 mm/day (Barman et al., 1964; Saitok et al., 1969). The white hair in this young woman was 3·5 cm long ± 0·3 cm; hence, the change in the host/tumour relationship occurred 78 ± 6·6 days before the photograph. Careful scrutiny of her clinical history did not reveal any apparent cause for the changed relationship between host and tumour and it must have occurred at least six to seven months before there were symptoms of advancing disease.

History and physical examination are typical for sizeable lymph node involvement. As a diagnostic test, lymphangiography initially seemed most promising as a means of establishing early invasion. However, my experience would be in accord with that reported by Cox (Cox et al., 1966), in which the test was shown to have too many false negatives and false positives to be sufficiently reliable as a means of determining the patient's future treatment. False negatives arise when the tumour completely fills the lymph nodes so that no lymph flows into it or when the injected lymphatic bypasses certain nodes. The false positives arise from small inclusions of fat or vascular pedicle in the hilar region of the lymph node.

Liver function tests do not appear to have a predictive value. Liver scans are performed as a routine and in future years it may be possible to give more precise assessment of their value. Suffice it to say at present that three patients who would have been considered incurable because of a positive liver scan but who had no other sign of disease have had a laparotomy performed and no sign of metastases was discovered. The X-ray features of bones have already been mentioned. Laparotomy is the only sure way of diagnosing intestinal or retroperitoneal metastases. Secondaries in the bladder can be visualised by the cystoscope or appear as filling defects in the bladder wall.

Ikonopisov (1972) felt happy that he was able to detect early dissemination of melanoma by a raised serum copper. However, a series of serum copper estimations done in my cases by my colleague Miss Blomfield (Milton and Blomfield, 1970) showed that although a raised serum copper does occur in advanced malignant melanoma, this is not sufficiently reliable to be of predictive value.

Dintenfass observed changes in blood viscosity in malignant disease and in a variety of other conditions (Dintenfass et al., 1966; Dintenfass and Sharp, 1969; Dintenfass and Bauer, 1970). Results of the study on viscosity factors in 43 patients with malignant melanoma indicated that there is an elevation of the viscosity factors in patients with the disease and that those who die from metastatic disease have a higher viscosity of the blood and of the plasma than patients who survive ($P > 0.001$). There was also a significant difference between patients who had A blood group and those who had O blood group in the aggregation of red cells in the viscosity of artificial thrombi ($P > 0.001$ and $P > 0.005$, respectively) (Dintenfass and Milton, 1973). Although these results are statistically significant, the explanation of them at the present time remains obscure. However, in future, viscosity factors may have an interest in terms of prognosis.

REFERENCES

Barman, J. M., Pecoraro, V. & Astore, I. (1964) Method, technic and computations in the study of the trophic state of the human scalp hair. *The Journal of Investigative Dermatology*, **42**, 421.

Clark, W. H., Jr, From, L., Bernadino, E. A., *et al.* (1969) The histogenesis and biologic behaviour of primary human malignant melanoma of the skin. *Cancer Research*, **29**, 705.

Cox, K. R., Hare, W. S. C. & Bruce, P. T. (1966) Lymphography in melanoma; correlation of radiology with pathology. *Cancer*, **19**, 637

Dintenfass, L. & Bauer, G. E. (1970) Dynamic blood coagulation and viscosity and degradation of artificial thrombi in patients with hypertension. *Cardiovascular Research*, **4**, 50.

Dintenfass, L., Julian, D. G. & Miller, G. E. (1966) Viscosity of blood in normal subjects and in patients suffering from coronary occlusion and arterial thrombosis. *American Heart Journal*, **71**, 587.

Dintenfass, L. & Milton, G. W. (1973) Blood viscosity factors and prognosis in malignant melanoma. *Medical Journal of Australia*, **1**, 1091.

Dintenfass, L. & Sharp, A. (1969) Dynamic blood coagulation, thrombus formation and degradation in patients with peripheral vascular disease (arteriosclerosis including diabetic): an *in vitro* study. *Annals of Surgery*, **170**, 984.

Ikonopisov, L. R. (1972) Non-biopsy diagnosis of malignant melanoma. In *Melanoma and Skin Cancer. Proceedings of the International Cancer Conference, Sydney, 1972*, ed. McCarthy, W. H., p. 223. Sydney: Government Printer.

Lewis, M. G. (1972) Immunological studies in patients with malignant melanoma: the role of circulating antibody. In *Melanoma and Skin Cancer. Proceedings of the International Cancer Conference, Sydney, 1972*, ed. McCarthy, W. H., p. 233. Sydney: Government Printer.

McLeod, G. R., Beardmore, G. L., Little, J. H., *et al.* (1971) Results of treatment of 361 patients with malignant melanoma in Queensland. *Medical Journal of Australia*, **1**, 1211.

Milton, G. W. (1963) Some methods used in the management of metastatic malignant melanoma. *Australasian Journal of Dermatology*, **7**, 15.

Milton, G. W. & Blomfield, Jeanette (1970) Serum copper studies in melanoma. Proceedings of the Surgical Research Society of Australasia. *Australian and New Zealand Journal of Surgery*, **39**, 317.

Milton, G. W., McCarthy, W. H. & Carlon, Anne (1971) Malignant melanoma and vitiligo. *The Australasian Journal of Dermatology*, **12**, 131.

Saitok, M., *et al.* (1969) *Advances in Biology of Skin IX: Hair Growth*, ed. Montagna, W. & Dobson, R. L., p. 183. Oxford: Pergamon.

Stephenson, E. M., Stephenson, N. G. & Milton, G. W. (1973) Unpublished data.

9. Treatment of Metastases

The care of the patient with secondary melanoma will be described under the following headings:

1. Potentially curable disease.
2. Definitely incurable disease.
3. Palliative, symptomatic or investigative methods of treatment.

POTENTIALLY CURABLE DISEASE

Definition of objectives of treatment

Potentially curable secondary disease implies a fit patient without clinical or other evidence of recurrence beyond the immediate vicinity of the site of the primary tumour or the draining lymph nodes, i.e. no evidence of blood borne metastasis. The thoughtful approach to such a patient takes the following factors into account. The disease, once it has recurred, is dangerous. Although the prognosis for most local recurrence is bad, it is not hopeless. Surgical treatment is admittedly mechanistic, but the result of treatment of metastasis by other methods is not encouraging. An otherwise fit patient in a potentially lethal situation should be offered surgical excision, even if this is extensive, as long as there are reasonable grounds for believing the condition is curable. However, the patients who have a short life expectancy from other causes, such as age, can often be managed by non-operative means (p. 89). Any patient who declines surgery can, of course, be cared for by the same non-operative techniques. Each day of normal healthy life is precious to anyone in this plight so it is important to limit hospitalisation to the minimum.

Recurrence in the scar

Recurrence in the scar of the primary lesion is treated by wide excision and skin graft in the manner described on page 48. If there was no lymph node resection as part of the first operation, the line of spread is taken as the axis of excision, but if the lymph nodes have been resected, and especially if the limb is oedematous, the excision of recurrences is circular and centres on the recurrence.

It is wise to discuss with the patient the necessity for carrying out a prophylactic node dissection if this has not been done, because it has been shown that the deeper the primary disease extends into the dermis, the greater the chance of dissemination, and it follows that nodal spread is likely after subcutaneous recurrence at the primary site. I must admit this is an opinion, and the figures at present available are not adequate proof that lymphatic involvement is certain under these circumstances.

INTRANSIT RECURRENCES

These are treated by excision as the first step, with or without lymphadenectomy.

RECURRENCE IN THE REGIONAL LYMPH NODES

Recurrence here or in the vicinity of the nodes is a surgical problem and lymph node dissection must be meticulous, or there is a danger of recurrence in the scar.

RECURRENT DISEASE AT THE SITE OF PREVIOUS LYMPH NODE DISSECTION

One of the more distressing aspects of recurrent melanoma is the tendency for the disease to recur at operation sites. With the operations described (Chs. 5, 6 and 7), the local recurrence rate is very low. After more limited procedures, local recurrence of the disease is probably more likely; precise figures are very difficult to obtain. However, many patients are sent to the clinic having had initial surgery elsewhere, once the disease has recurred close to the operation site. It is not possible to relate the pattern of recurrence to any specific detail of surgical technique, because the operations have been done by a variety of surgeons and the techniques varied. However, a pattern of recurrent disease at operation sites emerges:

Cervical recurrence

Recurrence after a radical dissection of glands in the neck usually occurs under the flaps and not on the margin of the wound and appears to be distributed almost randomly in the area of the dissection (the excised nodes have often been free of microscopic tumour deposits). If these metastases are left untreated, their progressive enlargement causes extremely distressing and enormous growths in the neck (Fig. 9.1). If recurrence in the neck is diagnosed while the lesions are smaller than 0·75 cm, intralesional injections of Thiotepa is the first method of treatment and this is followed by antigens and other chemotherapeutic agents (p. 89), as long as the agents are effective. However, once intralesional chemotherapy is ineffective, as shown by a progressively enlarging mass, it is no use to procrasti-

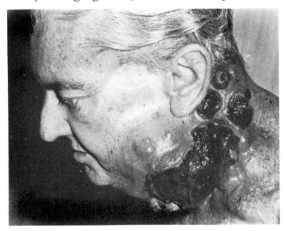

Fig. 9.1 Shows the enormous local recurrence of malignant melanoma at the site of a previous radical neck dissection. The original lymph nodes did not contain tumour.

nate by using radiotherapy or other therapeutic measures. I believe that first choice in the treatment at this stage consists of a surgical re-excision. Such an excision does not cure the patient, but avoids the considerable distress of massive local disease.

Axillary recurrence

There are three common sites of recurrence of malignant melanoma in a previously dissected axilla.

1. Commonest is probably the apex of the axilla proximal to the highest point reached by the previous dissection (Fig. 9.2).

2. Another point of recurrence is in the scar of the previous operation, whether this is a formal excision or a biopsy.

3. The site of previous drainage tubes (Fig. 9.3).

In elderly patients, small isolated nodules developing in an axilla are probably best treated with intralesional chemotherapy (p. 89). Only if this fails should recourse be made to surgical excision. In view of the investigative nature of intralesional chemotherapy in people of younger age groups it is probably wise to carry out surgical excision as the first method of definitive treatment.

The characteristic of malignant melanoma to displace tissue rather than invade it is valuable when a secondary dissection of the axilla is contemplated. Recurrence of tumour at the apex of the axilla is not usually in the previous operative field because the commonest failure in axillary dissection is to leave the apex intact. The diagnosis of an apical axillary mass can often be made by the fact that as the tumour enlarges it pushes the pectoralis major forward so the line of the chest below the clavicle becomes convex (Fig. 9.2). Large masses of this type may be removed once the tissue plane between the tumour and axilla vessels and nerves has been identified.

Groin recurrence

The three common sites of recurrent disease close to an inguinal node dissection are:

1. The external iliac lymph node immediately above the inguinal ligament. The

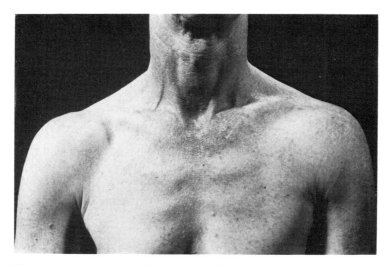

Fig. 9.2   This patient had previously had a 'radical' dissection of the left axillary lymph nodes.
Note: (1) Recurrent disease high in the axilla above the previous operation. (2) The scar of the original operation is not visible because the dissection was done entirely from below.

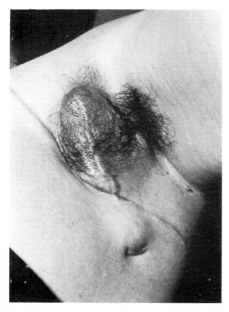

Fig. 9.3   Two common sites of recurrent disease after axillary dissection.
Note: (1) Recurrent tumour in the scar of a previous biopsy done to establish the diagnosis. (2) Recurrent tumour at the site of a drainage tube.

diagnosis of this is established by a lump detected at this point.

2. A mass close to the scar of the original operation, usually just below the inguinal ligament in the upper part of the scar. The clinical features of this are of an enlarging mass in the area.

3. Single, but more frequently multiple, small recurrences just distal to the scar and close to the line of spread. These recurrences are in the major lymphatic trunks of the thigh and they first appear at the site described above. As the disease extends, the tumour masses permeate the lymphatics of the thigh until almost all subcutaneous tissues of the region are packed with black growing tumour (Fig. 9.4).

The most important feature of the treatment of inguinal recurrence is to detect it early. If the mass is above the inguinal ligament, excision of the iliac lymph nodes is a straightforward procedure. Those in the scar and in the major lymphatics can, at an early stage, be removed by a re-do of the original operation taking a wider area and grafting the defect. It is very important that any secondary excision in the thigh is done with extreme thoroughness and over a broad width; otherwise further

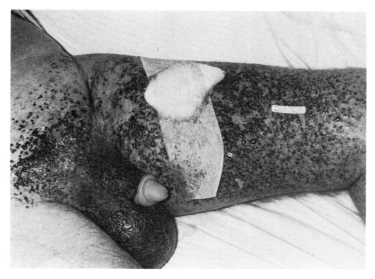

Fig. 9.4   Melanoma *en cuirasse*, which occurs after the disease develops close to a failed groin dissection if the extending tumour is left untreated and the patient does not die from generalised dissemination.

recurrence in the second operation site is almost inevitable. If recurrence does occur after an attempted ablation, then the lesions can often be controlled by intralesional injections provided, as always, the lesions are diagnosed when they are less than 0·75 cm in diameter p. 89).

For limbs in which the subcutaneous tissues have been massively replaced by melanoma, isolated limb perfusion may be tried if the operator is experienced with it; but it is usually preferable, if the patient is young and has good general health and the disease appears to be confined to the lymph glands, to consider seriously a high amputation (p. 91) or the Hueston procedure (p. 88), followed by systemic chemotherapy or immunotherapy.

Isolated limb perfusion

Isolated limb perfusion of the extremities for malignant melanoma was introduced in 1966 by Creech and Krementz because the limiting factor in the use of most chemotherapeutic agents is their toxic effect on normal tissues, especially the haemopoietic tissues and the gut mucosa. The effectiveness of the treatment will depend on four factors:

1. The action of the agent or agents used on the tumour.

2. The damage these agents may cause the normal tissues.

3. The completeness of the isolation of the limb.

4. The extent to which the tumour is confined to the limb.

1. If a chemotherapeutic agent could be developed that would be as effective against tumour cells and as harmless to normal cells as the antibiotics are effective in their action against bacteria and harmless to host tissues, the need for both ablative surgery and techniques like isolated limb perfusion would disappear overnight. However, such an agent does not yet exist, so isolated limb perfusion has been extensively investigated. The agents used fall into two categories—chemotherapeutic and heat, or a combination of the two. The commonest agents used have been phenylalanine mustard (melphalan) (Golomb *et al.*, 1962; Cox, Hare and Bruce, 1966; Stehlin, Giovanella and de Ipolyi, 1975) and thiotepa (Cox *et al.*, 1966). Cavaliere *et al.* (1967) used heat without adjunctive chemotherapy. Cox *et al.* (1966) and Stehlin (1969) combined both

heat and a chemotherapeutic agent during perfusion.

Golomb et al. (1962) described how, within a few days, visible tumour deposits begin to soften, liquefy and eventually dry up and become scaly, and small nodules began to leave depigmented patches in the skin. The same type of response (only slower) occurs after effective systemic chemotherapy (p. 99). The type of response does not appear to be influenced by the agent used. Cox et al. (1966) pointed out, I believe correctly, that any 'single shot' therapy is unlikely to kill all the tumour cells, and failure to do so may delay but not prevent recurrence of the disease.

2. Damage to the normal tissues of the limb by perfusion had been recorded by most authors (Creech and Krementz, 1966; Cox et al., 1966; Stehlin, 1969) and includes arterial thrombosis, gross persistent oedema and peripheral nerve injury. If these effects are severe, the patient has an added burden to carry.

3. If the perfused limb is not totally isolated from the remainder of the patient's circulation, severe toxic effects can occur; to prevent this, Stehlin et al. (1960), Golomb et al. (1962) and Cox et al. (1966) all used markers of different types in the perfusate which could be identified if they escaped above the tourniquet. All authors quoted above agree that both the local and general ill-effects of isolated limb perfusion can be reduced to a small proportion of the cases treated, provided the technique is meticulous. This treatment is, therefore, one for a special unit and not for the occasional operator.

4. The value of isolated limb perfusion in terms of patient survival must depend on the extent to which the malignant melanoma is confined to one limb, and this in turn will be influenced by the stage at which the treatment is performed. The protagonists of the technique write favourably of the survival figures (Creech et al., 1958; Golomb et al., 1962; Stehlin et al., 1975; Rochlin and Smart, 1965; Krementz and Ryan, 1972). Cox (1974 and 1975) felt that overall survival might not be greatly influenced by isolated limb perfusion, although local destruction of tumour in a limb

was often spectacular. He also reported that the survival of men was worse than that of women, a common finding with all methods of treatment for malignant melanoma. One may summarise the place of isolated limb perfusion in the treatment of malignant melanoma by the following:

1. In the hands of experts, the treatment is favourably reported.

2. In inexpert hands it is dangerous.

3. Its true place in treatment is still *sub judice*.

4. The event of more effective agents, of immunotherapy or of more careful use of intralesional therapy may render this elaborate technique unnecessary.

My personal experience is limited to six patients on whom the treatment has been tried and the results were equivocal, so I would not wish to venture a definite opinion on the method.

Integumentectomy

Hueston (1970) described the operation of integumentectomy, i.e. excision of all or nearly all the skin, subcutaneous tissue, and deep fascia of the limb on the understanding that spreading melanoma from the periphery does not penetrate the intact deep fascia. The operation requires very large free grafts and can be used as an alternative to amputation as the indications for it are similar. In carefully selected cases it can be a very useful procedure. The criteria for selection are: (1) the disease is confined to the limb; (2) the disease is too extensive in the limb to be controlled by intralesional injections (p. 89); (3) the patient has not had multiple or extensive excisions of previous recurrent melanoma in the limb, thereby breaching the deep fascia at several points. One disadvantage of integumentectomy is that it may require prolonged (4 to 6 weeks) hospitalisation for a patient who has a short life expectancy. I have performed this operation four times; in three, the disease recurred either in the limb or then systemically and the patients died. One case remains well and free of disease four years after integumentectomy.

Amputation

Major amputation is rarely advised as a treatment for malignant melanoma; the patients for whom it is recommended will be considered on page 91, where its place in palliation will be discussed.

DEFINITELY INCURABLE DISEASE

Definition of objectives of treatment

Malignant melanoma frequently differs from other malignant tumours by becoming incurable while the patient remains well. It is not reasonable to discuss results of treatment of such patients in terms of five-year survival, but the unpleasant word 'salvage' crops up, as indeed some patients with advanced malignant melanoma do survive. Once the hope of cure has vanished the philosophical approach to the patient changes. Extensive ablative surgery is only justified to relieve definite symptoms and even then it should be kept to a minimum. Every day or week in hospital represents a large proportion of the patient's remaining useful life, hence hospitalisation must be brief. Pain, suffering and expense incurred by the patient can no longer be justified by the hope of long-term benefits. The purpose of treatment, therefore, is speedy relief of present symptoms.

Intralesional chemotherapy

Eighty-eight patients with incurable melanoma have been treated by intralesional injections of one or more agents into tumour nodules. The objective of this treatment is to eliminate or reduce the nodules of recurrent tumour. Indications for intralesion injection are:

1. The patient must have proven disseminated melanoma beyond the field of local recurrence or decline, or be unsuitable for excisional therapy for other reasons, e.g. old age.

2. The patient must be in good general health.

3. The nodules must be easily accessible and the injections done as an outpatient procedure.

4. The skin over the lumps should be intact because the injected material will leak through the surface of a fungating lesion.

5. The lesion to be injected should be as small as possible, less than *2 cm diameter*, preferably less than 1 cm, because this treatment is ineffective with larger lesions.

6. It is important *not* to repeat injecting the same substance into any one tumour nodule. If the injected nodule enlarges apparently unaffected by the treatment, there is no point in using the same agent a second time; if it does not enlarge, or diminishes, the same injection is repeated two or possibly three times and the injected material is then changed.

7. The chemotherapeutic agent is dissolved in the smallest volume of sterile water or saline sufficient to dissolve it, preferably less than 1·5 ml. The best syringe is a 1 ml tuberculin syringe, and care must be taken to exclude air bubbles or the agent may leak into the subcutaneous tissues while the needle is being withdrawn from the tumour mass (Table 9.1). The

Table 9.1   Intralesional therapy

Agent	Dosage (mg)
Trenimon[a]	0·2
Nitrogen mustard	20
Thiotepa (Lederle)	15–30
Phenylalanine mustard—	
Melphalan (Burrows Welcome)	up to 50
Methotrexate (Lederle)	10
BCG[b]	up to 75

[a]An alkylating agent formerly manufactured by Bayers Pharmaceutical.
[b]Theiss or Pasteur strain prepared by Commonwealth Serum Laboratories, Victoria, Australia.

method of injection is to place the agent directly in the centre of the small tumour mass by fixing the nodule with the index finger and thumb of the left hand. The needle is inserted through the skin some distance from the mass and passes through the subcutaneous tissues before entering it. The patient is reviewed in two weeks and if the lump has remained the same size or become smaller, the dose is repeated; if it has enlarged, another agent is chosen. However, if the nodule fails to show response after three or four injections, no further direct assaults on it by injection are made. It is important not to overdo the injections at any one site because an unpleasant slough can be caused by excessive local chemotherapy, especially with nitrogen mustard and Trenimon (Fig. 9.5). A single lymph node or isolated nodule can, in about 70 per cent of cases, be either considerably reduced in size or become completely impalpable following repeated injections of one or more agents. This diminution in size has not been followed for prolonged periods because such patients have a limited life expectancy, but there have been four elderly people (80+) who had complete disappearance of palpable metastatic lymph nodes. The palpable node did not return for periods up to 18 months by which time these patients died from other causes, the disease had spread elsewhere, or the patient remained well.

8. The chemotherapeutic agent is presumably rapidly absorbed into the general circulation, but as the injections are infrequent, no systemic effects have been observed.

9. In a patient who has more than one subcutaneous metastasis, it is tempting to try different agents in each of the lesions and in this way ascertain which chemotherapeutic agent will be most effective when used by systemic administration. I have attempted to do this on eight occasions but unfortunately the results do not appear to have any predictive value. Of the 88 patients treated with intralesional chemotherapy, the best tumour regression was obtained following the use of thiotepa or BCG. Nitrogen mustard caused central necrosis of tumour deposits, but a viable and growing shell of tumour always remained around the periphery. Methotrexate was ineffective in reducing or restraining tumour growth in five out of six cases. Both nitrogen mustard and methotrexate are now used only if other methods fail. Our results are not adequate to make a definitive statement concerning the effect of intralesional therapy on the survival of the patient, and for the present this method of treatment is considered palliative. The regression of injected nodules is 62·5 per cent of those injected, but one cannot predict which lesion will respond because different tumour nodules respond differently to the same drug. Indeed, it has been frequently observed that if the same drug is used on two deposits in the same

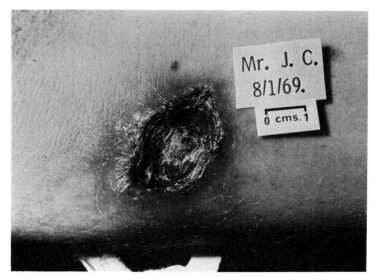

Fig. 9.5   Shows the unpleasant slough caused by repeated injection of an alkylating agent (Trenimon) into a subcutaneous nodule of melanoma.
Note: It is unwise to inject repeatedly the same agent into tumour deposits if it is ineffective in reducing the size of the lesion.

patient, one of the deposits may regress while the other continues to grow.

Topical chemotherapy

Topical chemotherapy on non-resectable fungating lesions: the circumstances which require this method of treatment are, fortunately, rare but some relief can be obtained from the distressing haemorrhage and discharge by the topical application of cytostatic cream with or without copper sulphate powder to small fungating tumours. The cream used is made up of methotrexate and Colcemid (methotrexate 9·5 per cent, Colcemid 0·5 per cent and Cucerin base). The cream should be applied in small quantities daily with a gloved finger and worked slowly into the raw surface of the tumour. A thin film of cream is placed on a dressing which covers the area. If the lesion continues to proliferate in spite of this treatment for three weeks, then the exuberant growth can be reduced by adding $CuSO_4$ ground to a fine powder and applied to the fungating surface before the cream. This method has been used in five cases in whom no other form of control appeared feasible. In each case the overgrown tissues became flattened, the discharge lessened but the lesion did not heal (Figs. 9.6 and 9.7). Fungating nodules can also be excised with a 1 cm margin of normal skin, and local recurrence in the scar is not inevitable in patients with a short life expectancy. Another agent sometimes useful in reducing fungating nodules is thiotepa (15 mg) dusted on as a powder once a week.

Excision

Palliative excision of small subcutaneous or lymph node metastases may be considered where the evidence of generalised dissemination is unsure. The excision then both constitutes therapy of the local lesion and proves the diagnosis. It is unnecessary to continue to excise all the recurrent nodules which appear once the diagnosis of general dissemination has been established, because they can be more easily controlled by intralesional cytostatic drug injection (p. 89) or by systemic chemotherapy (p. 99).

Very large or fungating deposits of melanoma may be excised as palliative treatment and with modest success, provided certain criteria are met:

1. The patient is anxious for relief and requests excision of the mass.
2. The patient's life expectancy is three months or so.
3. The discomfort of the operation and its sequelae are considered less distressing than the symptoms caused by the metastases.
4. No other non-operative method of treatment can be expected to offer the patient comparable relief.

The pathological difference between the invasiveness of melanoma and other cancers has been mentioned on page 81, and even large secondary lesions do not usually become attached to surrounding structures. Hence, provided the surgeon dissects on a plane deep to the lesion, he can usually resect the deposit without damage to major vessels or nerves. However, an exception to this rule occurs if the lesion is a recurrence in a previously operated field. In these circumstances, the growing tumour may envelop major structures in the vicinity and resection may be very difficult or impossible.

Amputation

Major amputation as a means of palliation has never been undertaken lightly but there have been 10 patients in this series in whom major amputation was carried out for palliation. In seven cases there was no proof of generalised dissemination of the disease so there was a faint chance of cure, but this was not used to persuade the patient to accept the operation. Eight hindquarter amputations have been done for repeated and uncontrollable recurrent disease in a leg; five were men and three women. None had evidence of central disease, but the extent of the local lesion implied that disease must be generalised. Of the men, three died between 9 and 18 months after amputation, two of these remained well and at work until a few weeks before death from cerebral recurrence, and one developed recurrent disease at the amputation site from

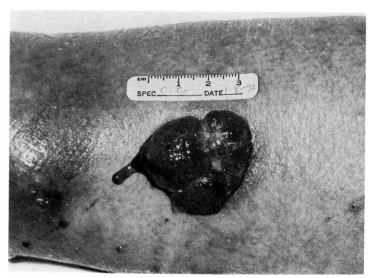

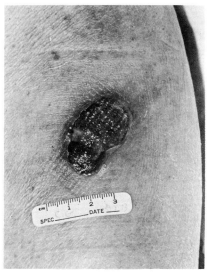

Figs. 9.6 and 9.7   Show the effect of Cytostatic cream with CuSO$_4$ applied for 28 days to a fungating metastasis in an 82-year-old woman who refused all other treatment.

which he obtained temporary relief with DTIC (p. 99). The two other men are still alive and well, one two years and the other five months after amputation. Two out of three women died from central disease less than one year after amputation and the third, who had the most extensive disease of all, remains in excellent health 14 years after amputation. One of the best descriptions of an operation in surgical literature is that of hindquarter amputation by Sir Gordon Gordon-Taylor, Craft and Jones (1955) and I could not add to that account regarding this operation except in so far as it is done for extensive melanoma in the leg. However, the following points emerge from the cases reported here:

1. Oedema associated with recurrent disease in the leg may be quite extensive, but fortunately it does not usually extend high on the *posterior* aspect of the thigh towards the

buttock. Both the skin flaps should be free of oedema; otherwise recurrence in the flap seems likely.

2. A totally non-oedematous posterior flap may be too short for closure without tension; if so, a split skin graft on the remaining defect will be adequate for the first 12 months; then a prosthesis can be considered.

3. The posterior flap must be thick as Gordon-Taylor *et al.* (1955) described or the upper inner edge may slough. If this happens, the slough should be immediately excised and the defect closed with a split skin graft.

4. A non-residue diet and full bowel preparation (including lavage) will allow the patient many postoperative days free of bowel movement.

5. Small local recurrences in the flaps should be immediately excised or injected (p. 85).

Radiotherapy

Radiotherapy has a limited place in the treatment of melanoma, but the tumour is often not as resistant to X-rays as is usually believed. The principles which govern the use of radiotherapy in melanoma (apart from Hutchinson's melanotic freckle) are that the tumour to be treated should be small and the blood supply to the area good. When these criteria apply, a large dose of radiation can be administered and the amount of tumour regression may be very gratifying (see bone pain below).

Management of pain

Malignant melanoma is usually a painless disease; however, under some circumstances the disease may cause considerable pain.

Bone secondaries may be very painful and it is fortunate that this is relieved by radiotherapy with the same facility as localised bone pain caused by other types of metastasis. Indeed, if the pain has not diminished within a week of commencing treatment, the pain is not due to bone metastasis. The remarkable easing of bone pain by radiotherapy when the tumour itself may be resistant to the effects of X-rays suggests at least two speculations. Either melanoma in bone is more sensitive to irradiation than elsewhere (not likely because the bones usually do not recalcify), or the relief of bone pain depends on the effect of the ray on the normal tissues in bone and not on the tumour response. Metastases in the region of the spine often involve nerve roots and the only effective treatment is decompression. This can be an important step in any case because the rapid development of paraplegia may follow nerve root compression (p. 80). Pain from fungating and infected lesions is best treated by dealing directly with the lesion itself (p. 91).

Pain occurring in the terminal stages of the disease requires continuous use of analgesics (Milton, 1972). It is an advantage if the medication can be given orally so that the patient remains at home; however, if the patient is hospitalised, in pain and has only a few weeks to live, morphine should be used in large and regular doses adequate to bring the patient mental and physical rest. A patient should always be allowed to request and receive supplemental analgesics if the pain returns before the next regular analgesic is due.

PALLIATIVE, SYMPTOMATIC OR INVESTIGATIVE METHODS OF TREATMENT

This chapter has so far been concerned with either easily accessible or fairly well localised metastatic melanoma. However, as the disease advances and dissemination becomes wider and deeper, some form of systemic treatment may be attempted which has three objectives:

1. To diminish the patient's suffering.
2. To prolong the patient's worthwhile life.
3. To try to find out which methods of treatment might achieve the first two objectives.

Symptomatic treatment

The objective of this treatment is to relieve symptoms and cause the patient minimum inconvenience. I will not go into any detail because the drugs are standard.

LIVER

The most prominent symptom of liver metastasis is nausea. Almost every known antiemetic has been tried and it cannot be claimed that any particular agent is more effective than the rest. Although oral antiemetics are frequently used, sooner or later the symptoms become so severe that the drug must be injected. It must be pointed out that nausea from liver metastasis is hard to check and it is wise to try maximum doses of a variety of antiemetics on each patient. The most frequently used antiemetics have been Maxolon (metoclopramide, Beecham) 10 mg, or Stemetil (prochlorperazine, May and Baker) 5–10 mg, both used three to four times daily.

CEREBRAL METASTASES

Cerebral metastases are of two kinds. Usually the deposits are multiple and scattered randomly throughout the brain; less frequently the metastasis may be or appear to be solitary. A solitary cerebral metastasis is best excised, if this is feasible, and followed-up with radiotherapy and chemotherapy (see below). Multiple metastases in the brain can be treated symptomatically (to relieve the headache), with aspirin and dexamethazone. This is supplemented with radiotherapy and chemotherapy (Beresford, 1969; Gottlieb, Frei and Luce, 1972; Hilaris *et al.*, 1963; Pennington and Milton, 1975). Newer forms of chemotherapy, such as methyl CCNU, may prove useful in the treatment of cerebral metastases. Large doses of the older chemotherapeutic agents such as phenylalanine mustard may be dangerous for patients with cerebral secondaries because the combination of a low platelet count and necrotic tumour often results in massive cerebral haemorrhage.

PULMONARY METASTASES

These are best treated with systemic DTIC (p. 99), but the dry, irritating cough they cause can often be relieved with noremethadone HCl, racemic-p-hydroxyephedrine Ticarda (Hoechst) 10 mg, in increasing doses up to 12 per 24 hours.

PLEURAL EFFUSION

This is best treated by aspiration and inserting a cytotoxic agent into the pleural cavity. The agents used have been the same as for drug-intratumour injections and the doses are the same (p. 89). The response to these drugs is capricious and in some patients the pleural effusion has been eliminated for prolonged periods, in others the reaccumulation appears to be uninfluenced by any of the drugs used.

ASCITES

Ascites from metastatic melanoma is treated by the same technique applied to the peritoneum as those used for pleural effusion (see above). Severe and recurrent haemoperitoneum may be associated with ascites and is virtually untreatable. Peritoneal lavage via a dialysis catheter using cytostatic agents has been tried on several occasions but has not arrested the bleeding.

Immunotherapy

Investigative methods of treatment include immunotherapy and chemotherapy. The background and results of immunotherapy have been reviewed in detail by Lewis *et al.* (Ch. 10), and I have added a few general observations (p. 138). Here I shall refer to the Sydney Hospital Melanoma Clinic's experience of immunotherapy in the treatment of advanced malignant melanoma.

SPECIFIC IMMUNE STIMULATION

The technique of obtaining irradiated tumour cells for injection was to remove an easily accessible metastasis, e.g. subcutaneous nodule, which was then placed in buffered Hanks Solution with penicillin and streptomycin. The tumour cells were squashed out of the nodule by splitting it in half and gently pressing it on a dish in a thin layer of the solution. Roughly 15 ml of cell suspension was obtained. The cell suspension was then irradiated with 12 000 rad. The patient was given regular intradermal injections of the suspension once every three weeks. None of the 14 patients treated by this method showed any detectable improvement or alteration to the course of their disease; the method was, therefore, abandoned.

The second method used at the clinic was to couple the patient's tumour cells to a highly antigenic protein, goat gamma globulin, using bisdiazo benzidine as a coupling agent. The method is described in detail by McCarthy *et al.* (1973) and Czajkowski *et al.* (1967). The hope of this method of treatment is that the weak antigens present on the surface of melanoma cells may be made more easily detectable by the host's defences if he is given the same tumour cell with a powerful antigen attached to them. It is hoped that the mechanisms will then produce a type of hypersensitivity by the host to the tumour.

the specific immunotherapy suggests the following conclusions:

1. The smaller the amount of tumour present the better the chance of improving the host's ability to reject the remaining tumour.

2. Patients with rapidly declining health will rarely obtain worthwhile benefit from immunotherapy.

3. The progress of the melanoma after immunotherapy is altered sufficiently often to be reasonably certain that there is a cause and effect relationship between the immunotherapy and the regression of the disease.

4. The type of metastatic melanoma which appears to be most vulnerable to the stimulated host's immune mechanism is the small intracu-

Table 9.2 The results obtained from using immunotherapy in patients with advanced melanoma. Specific immunotherapy = irradiated cells or coupled cells. Non-specific immunotherapy = virus or BCG

Type	No. of patients	Objective remission	Long-term remission	% remission
Irradiated cells	14	—	—	—
Coupled cells	76	10	4	14
Virus	66	13	2[a]	9
BCG[b]	30	—	—	—

[a]Nine years and 3 years.
[b]These patients will be considered separately (see Table 9.3).

The results of this method of treatment in our hands was more encouraging than using irradiated cells alone (Table 9.2). Four patients showed a long-term remission and of these four one remains alive now five years after the immunotherapy; the other three died at periods ranging between three to five years following treatment. In other words, the results of immunotherapy are those of very modest success but it is nevertheless a method of treatment which is highly desirable to investigate fully in case the results can be improved. An observation made on three occasions was the diminution of several metastases in one patient with a coincidental rapid growth of one or two other metastases in the same patient. This finding tends to support the idea that metastasising melanoma may be a polyclonal tumour and the separate clones have a different relationship to the host. Our experience with

taneous nodule or the small metastasis in the subcutaneous tissues. Large deposits in the lungs, and even more so in the liver, appear resistant to immune attack.

NON-SPECIFIC IMMUNE STIMULATION

VIRUS THERAPY

A total of 80 patients have been treated by inoculation of tumour deposits with vaccinia virus and the first case treated by this means was in 1959 (Belisario and Milton, 1961; Milton and Lane Brown, 1966). The virus used is attenuated smallpox vaccine BP (Commonwealth Serum Laboratories), i.e. vaccinia virus. The dose is difficult to determine with precision because the viability of the vaccinia varies slightly and the quantity of living organisms in any small volume may also vary. However, a dosage of up to 500 times the usual vaccination dose has been used, the average dose being approximately 100 vaccination doses.

It is important when administering vaccinia virus therapy to be sure that certain precautions are carefully observed. All members of the nursing staff who deal with these patients, their clothing or their bedding, must have been recently vaccinated. Nurses must be warned of the extreme danger of contaminating their eyes from the vaccinia or from discharge from the patient's pustules. The patient himself must be carefully supervised to see that he does not contaminate his own cornea.

Viral encephalitis has been reported following vaccination, but this is apparently not dose-related because there has been no suggestion of it in this series.

The type of metastases most suitable for treatment of direct inoculation of vaccinia virus is a metastasis in or close to the skin. I have not observed satisfactory results with any tumour deposits deeper than the draining lymph nodes, and in my experience liver and pulmonary metastases are unresponsive to vaccinia therapy, although Burdick (1960) did report some improvement in a case of his.

The method of treatment has been to inoculate directly all detectable tumour deposits with vaccinia virus. If the deposits are in the skin this can be done by scarification or multiple punctures; if the deposits are deeper then the vaccinia virus is inoculated by direct injection into the centre of the tumour mass. It is important while injecting to have available adrenalin and hydrocortisone in case of anaphylactic reaction. However, none of these patients have had any sign of anaphylaxis during treatment. If there are a large number of intracutaneous deposits then the patient may be given a short anaesthetic; however, if the lesions are few anaesthesia is unnecessary.

The immediate result of inoculating a large dose of virus into a patient is a febrile reaction within 12 hours of inoculation. This subsides in a matter of a few hours and is presumably the result of reaction to foreign protein. Four or five days after the inoculation, if the patient develops a good reaction, the lesions and surrounding skin become intensely inflamed with a typical pustular eruption. On five occasions the patients have developed generalised vaccinia pustules, which consist of a few, usually not more than half a dozen, pustules in distant parts of the body. In each of these cases the condition subsided with general nursing measures and no active treatment was required. In five patients an attempt was made to enhance the effect of vaccination by pre-treating the patient with prednisone. The prednisone increased the violence of the viral damage but did not appear to enhance the oncolytic effect. If the inoculated tumour deposits are going to regress following the vaccinia therapy, the first evidence that they will do so appears as the inflammatory reaction to the virus begins to subside. At this point, the tumour nodule which was formerly firm and convex becomes flattened and even concave as the inflammation gradually disappears over a period of five or six days following the initial inflammatory response (Figs. 9.8, 9.9, 9.10 and 9.11). If the patient has recently been vaccinated or is for other reasons immune to the effect of vaccinia and has no systemic or local reaction to the inoculation, I have not seen an instance in which the tumour showed any worthwhile regression. It follows from this that if the initial treatment with vaccinia is ineffective it is likely that subsequent treatments will also be ineffective and the agent, therefore, is not repeated.

Conclusions

1. The response of the tumour to vaccinia inoculation is too frequent to be a chance event, i.e. there must be a cause and effect relationship between inoculation with virus and regression of tumour.

2. Virus therapy has no place if the disease is distributed with massive central deposits.

3. The small localised cutaneous deposits in non-immune patients, the destruction of the tumour by virus inoculation, is better than 50 per cent, although prolonged survival is very much lower, i.e. about 5 per cent.

4. It appears that the virus effects may have a two-fold mechanism although this remains a speculation. The first mechanism is the local

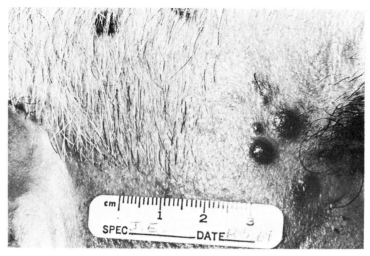

Fig. 9.8   The untreated metastases.

Figs. 9.8 to 9.11   Show the right side of the face in a man of 58 who developed blood borne intracutaneous metastases from a primary melanoma on the back, before and after vaccinia virus inoculation.

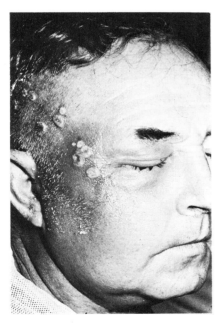

Fig. 9.9   The same lesions six days after they had been inoculated with vaccinia.

destructive power of the virus on the tumour cells, and the second is immune stimulation resulting from virus inoculation. It is unlikely that any virus will be sufficiently selective or sufficiently total in its oncolytic effects to be used as a 'magic bullet' or as an antibiotic.

5. It would be tempting to try to enhance the effect of viral oncolysis by one of several techniques. It might be possible, for example, to promote melanospecificity in vaccinia by repeated passage of virus through melanoma deposits in a series of patients. However, this has not been attempted because of the possibility of producing an alteration in virus, i.e. some form of mutation which could be extremely dangerous, e.g. such a virus might destroy the choroidal melanin.

6. The use of vaccinia virus in the treatment of advanced melanoma has a small but definite place in patients who have cutaneous deposits not responding to other methods of therapy, but it is by no means a method which can be regarded as proven beyond the point of being investigative. A recent report by Everall *et al.* (1975) has described the use of vaccinia in the treatment of primary malignant melanoma before excision. They report 25 cases in the

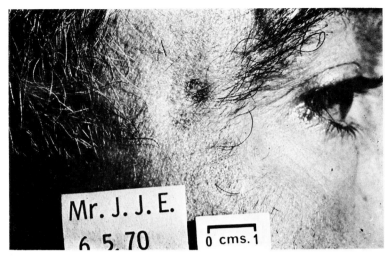

Fig. 9.10   One year later—pale, concave, pigmented scars remain, but no active tumour.

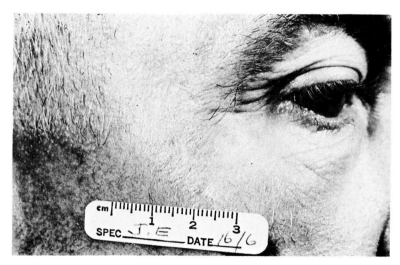

Fig. 9.11   Two years after treatment, there is no residual pigment.

initial result of this method which appears to be encouraging. However, it is my opinion that for the moment, once again, this method of treatment is still to be considered investigative.

BCG

Another non-specific immune stimulant under trial is *Baccilus Calmette-Guérin* (BCG) which has received considerable attention in relation to many tumours. Clinical experience with melanoma is confined to 19 patients who, between them, had 40 lesions treated by direct BCG inoculation into the lesion. Table 9.3 shows the results of this therapy. Permanent regression of treated lesions does occur and at a satisfactory rate, and similarly temporary regression of lesions is also frequently accomplished. However, it is still too soon to claim any conclusions which may be reached as regards the overall survival of these patients. Such methods of treatment are continually under review and it will be some years before the final place of BCG in the treatment of melanoma is established. However, at the present time BCG is useful in the destruction of local tumour deposits that do not respond to other methods of treatment, but it is now the practice of the clinic to excise any large lesions that have been treated with BCG at a stage when they are under regression. Another technique using BCG in the therapy of melanoma dealt with in some detail by Lewis et al. (Ch. 10, p. 131) is the use of cutaneous scarification of BCG not specifically in the tumour deposits. At present WHO is conducting a trial in the use of combined BCG and DTIC as a prophylactic for patients suffering from melanoma having a bad prognosis, and the results of this will be watched with great interest. At present, however, as with other forms of immunotherapy, it is still in the stage of investigation.

Table 9.3   The results of inoculation of BCG directly into metastatic tumour deposits

	Men	Women	Total
Permanent regression	6	2	8
Temporary regression	8	5	13
No change	5	5	10
Continued growth	5	4	9

Note: No. of patients = 19   No. of lesions treated = 40

Chemotherapy

Two methods of systemic chemotherapy which I have used will be considered:
1. The use of imidazole carboxamide (DTIC).
2. Triple therapy.

IMIDAZOLE CARBOXAMIDE (DTIC)
This agent was supplied by the Cancer Chemotherapy Division, National Service Centre, National Cancer Institute, U.S.A.

DTIC was used on a dose of 4·5 mg/kg body-weight by intravenous injection on 10 consecutive days. The patients were in hospital for the first two or three days of the treatment and then returned home to report back as an outpatient for the remaining injections. The daily injection of DTIC was preceded by an intravenous injection of Maxolon 10 mg and 1–2 Maxolon tablets given 4-hourly PRN for 8 to 12 hours after the injection. The patient's blood picture was checked before and at weekly intervals afterwards for the first two months. If the patient showed any response the course of DTIC was repeated. However, our initial experience (Burke, McCarthy and Milton, 1971) discouraged me from the value of multiple courses. Hence in recent years if one method of treatment has not produced any worthwhile results within eight weeks another is used.

Results

Side effects. Virtually all patients noticed an unpleasant nausea and vomiting commencing about $1\frac{1}{2}$ hours after the first injection and persisting for a few hours. The duration and severity of this is variable, but most patients class it as singularly unpleasant for the first and second injection; however, by the time the third or fourth injection is given the patient is usually not disturbed by nausea. Changes in the white cell count were variable and difficult to predict, but in no instance was there any serious or prolonged fall of the leukocyte count. Table 9.4 shows the improvement rates. Another effect of DTIC treatment which is difficult to quantify is the observation, especially by the nursing staff, that patients undergoing therapy are often severely emotionally depressed even to the extent of refusing further treatment.

Table 9.4   The number of patients and the results of treatment using the single agent DTIC (imidazole carboxamide) and triple therapy

Drug	No. of patients	Detectable remission	Long remission	% remission
DTIC	66	18	3	27
Triple	52	14	2	27

Comment

The effect of DTIC is encouraging in that it implies that effective chemotherapeutic agents are not beyond hope. The average duration of remission was measured in months with the exception of three patients in whom the disease had regressed for up to three years. I have not seen any patient in whom there appeared to be any possibility of a permanent cure.

TRIPLE THERAPY

As the name implies this method of chemotherapy uses three different agents in each patient. The study was part of a WHO chemotherapeutic trial for melanoma. Each patient was given one of two regimes (Table 9.5); if some tumour regression was observed the course was repeated in two months, a total of 55 courses being given.

Table 9.5   The two regimes for triple therapy used in the treatment of advanced melanoma

Regime I (27 patients)

Drug	Dosage	
DTIC	100 mg/m²	(days 1 to 5 inclusive)
BCNU	100 mg/m²	(day 1)
Vincristine	1·4 mg/m²	(days 1 and 15)

Regime II (25 patients)

Drug	Dosage	
DTIC	100 mg/m²	(days 1 to 5 inclusive)
BCNU	100 mg/m²	(day 1)
Dactinomycin	0·05 mg/kg	(days 1 and 15)

Results

The morbidity of the treatment was not severe except for nine cases of alopecia in patients on regime 1. There was no other significant difference detected between the two regimes (e.g. WBC). No patient on either regime survived for more than $3\frac{1}{2}$ years after treatment; both long-term remissions, i.e. 2 years or more, were in regime 2. The overall results of triple therapy were no better than those obtained when DTIC was used alone, and the morbidity from triple therapy was greater than that from DTIC. A full account of this trial was reported by Beretta *et al.*, 1976.

SUMMARY

When reviewing the different methods of treatment used for advanced malignant melanoma it seems as if a small proportion of patients (probably about 10 per cent) would have considerable and even lasting benefit from either immune, virus or chemotherapy. The factors which determine the response to these treatments are unknown, but as a rule small amounts of tumour, superficially situated, appear to have the best response. Presumably the factors which determine the pattern of spread are similar to those which render the tumour vulnerable to treatment. The obvious conclusion is that the subtleties of the host–tumour dialogue are a long way from being understood.

REFERENCES

Belisario, J. C. & Milton, G. W. (1961) The experimental local therapy of cutaneous metastases of malignant melanoblastomas with cow pox vaccine or colcemid (demecolcine or omaine). *Australian Journal of Dermatology*, **6**, 113.
Beresford, H. R. (1969) Melanoma of the nervous system. Treatment with corticosteroids and radiation. *Neurology*, **19**, 59.
Beretta, G., Bonadorma, G., Cascinelli, N., Morabito, A. & Veronesi, U. (1976) Comparative evaluation of three combination regimens for advanced melanoma. *Cancer Treatment Reports*, **60**, 33.
Burdick, K. H. (1960) Malignant melanoma treated with vaccinia injections. *Archives of Dermatology*, **82**, 438.
Burke, P. J., McCarthy, W. H. & Milton, G. W. (1971) Imidazole carboxamide therapy in advanced malignant melanoma. *Cancer*, **27**, 744.
Cavaliere, R., Ciogatto, E. C., Giovanella, B. C., *et al.* (1967) Selective heat sensitivity of cancer cells: biochemical and clinical studies. *Cancer*, **20**, 1351.
Cox, K. R. (1974) Regional cutaneous metastasis in melanoma of the limb. *Surgery, Gynecology and Obstetrics*, **139**, 385.
Cox, K. R. (1975) Survival after regional perfusion for limb melanoma. *Australian and New Zealand Journal of Surgery*, **45**, 32.

Cox, K. R., Hare, W. S. C. & Bruce, P. T. (1966) Lymphography in melanoma; correlation of radiology with pathology. *Cancer*, **19**, 637.

Creech, O., Jr. & Krementz, E. T. (1966) Techniques of regional perfusion. *Surgery*, **60**, 938.

Creech, O., Jr, Krementz, E. T., Ryan, F. R., *et al.* (1958) Chemotherapy of cancer: regional perfusion utilizing an extracorporeal circuit. *Annals of Surgery*, **148**, 616.

Czajkowski, N. P., Rosenblatt, M., Wolf, P. L., *et al.* (1967) A new method of active immunisation to autologous human tumour tissue. *Lancet*, ii, 905.

Everall, J. D., O'Doherty, C. J., Wand, J., *et al.* (1975) Treatment of primary melanoma by intralesional vaccinia before excision. *Lancet*, ii, 583.

Golomb, F. M., Postel, A. H., Hall, A. B., *et al.* (1962) Chemotherapy of human cancer by regional perfusion. Report of 52 perfusions. *Cancer*, **15**, 828.

Gordon-Taylor, G., Craft, A. W. J. & Jones, R. N. (1955) *Amputations in Modern Operative Surgery*. 4th edition, ed. Turner, G. & Rogers, L. C. London: Cassell.

Gottlieb, J. A., Frei, E. & Luce, J. K. (1972) An evaluation of the management of patients with cerebral metastases from malignant melanoma. *Cancer*, **29**, 701.

Hilaris, B. S., Raben, M., Calabrese, A. S., *et al.* (1963) Value of radiation therapy for distant metastases from malignant melanoma. *Cancer*, **16**, 765.

Hueston, J. T. (1970) Integumentectomy for malignant melanoma of the limbs. *Australian and New Zealand Journal of Surgery*, **40**, 114.

Krementz, E. T. & Ryan, F. R. (1972) Chemotherapy of melanoma of the extremities by perfusion: fourteen years clinical experience. *Annals of Surgery*, **175**, 900.

McCarthy, W. H., Kossard, S., Milton, G. W., *et al.* (1973) Immunotherapy of malignant melanoma: A clinical trial. *Cancer*, **32**, 97.

Milton, G. W. (1972) The care of the dying. *Medical Journal of Australia*, **2**, 177.

Milton, G. W. & Lane Brown, M. M. (1966) The limited role of attenuated smallpox virus in the management of advanced malignant melanoma. *Australian and New Zealand Journal of Surgery*, **35**, 286.

Pennington, D. G. & Milton, G. W. (1975) Cerebral metastasis from melanoma. *Australian and New Zealand Journal of Surgery*, **45**, 405.

Rochlin, D. B. & Smart, C. R. (1965) Treatment of malignant melanoma by regional perfusion. *Cancer*, **18**, 1544.

Stehlin, J. S. (1969) Hypothermic perfusion with chemotherapy for cancers of the extremities. *Surgery, Gynecology and Obstetrics*, **129**, 305.

Stehlin, J. S., Jr, Clark, R. J., Jr, Smith, J. L., Jr, *et al.* (1960) Malignant melanoma of the extremities: experiences with conventional therapy: a new surgical and chemotherapeutic approach with regional perfusion. *Cancer*, **13**, 55.

Stehlin, J. S., Giovanella, B. C., de Ipolyi, P. D., Muenz, L. R. & Anderson, R. F. (1975) Results of hyperthermic perfusion for melanoma of the extremities. *Surgery, Gynecology and Obstetrics*, **140**, 339.

10. Immunology and Immunotherapy of Malignant Melanoma

Martin G. Lewis

INTRODUCTION

The concept of immune reactivity in human tumours and its ultimate exploitation in immunotherapy is by no means new (Hamilton-Fairley, 1969). Nevertheless, advances over the last few years are beginning to make this a reality. The study of human malignant melanoma has played a major role in the elucidation of the complexities seen in the relationship between the immune system and the development of neoplasia (Lewis, 1974b; Nairn, 1974; Gutterman et al., 1975a). Much of the early laboratory-based work in the field of tumour immunology concentrated its force on understanding the rejection of transplanted or chemically induced tumours in rodents, and as such resulted in such terminologies as tumour-specific transplantation antigens (TSTA). The idea that individuals bearing tumours might respond immunologically had already been suggested before the turn of the century. During the past 10 years, evidence has indicated that individual patients can in fact mount a tumour-associated immune response, which may or may not be related to the transplantation or rejection antigens systems seen in syngeneic experimental animals. In this review of the subject, the emphasis will be placed on evidence for immune reactions in the individual patient against his own tumour and the possible mechanisms to explain why this initial immune response fails to control the spread of malignancy. In particular, metastatic spread in patients with malignant melanoma will be the major reference point. It is appropriate, therefore, that we start by considering some remarks

Note: This chapter was prepared with the assistance of Geoffrey Rowden and Terence M. Phillips.

made by Paul Ehrlich in a lecture in London in 1900, where he referred to the already established work of Von Dungen and other suggesting that antisera might be raised against squamous cell carcinomas and other carcinomas of the skin (Himmelweitt, 1957). Eve, in his lectures to general practitioners in 1903 on melanoma, pointed out the possibility of host factors playing important roles. An extensive study by Sampson Handley over a period of years, ranging from the turn of the century until 1907, showed clear evidence of lymphocytic infiltrates in malignant melanoma and suggested that this was a form of host rejection of the tumour. Over the next few years various contributions were added to these ideas, including the work of Coley and Hoguet (1916) with their interest in both spontaneous regression and the part played by certain bacterial infections in regression or arrest of malignancy.

Unfortunately, although these early years of the twentieth century produced tremendous enthusiasm in the field of immunotherapy following on the early observations and suggestions of the late nineteenth century, an era of pessimism developed in the wake of the lack of success. This was summarised by Woglom in 1929 in referring to tumour immunology as follows: 'Nothing may be hoped for at present in respect to a successful therapy in this direction'. Between that time and the establishment in the 1950s by Foley (1953), Prehn and Main (1957), Baldwin (1955) and others of tumour specific antigens in animals, the field of human tumour immunology died down to a very low ebb. The use of syngeneic inbred animal strains and the establishment that chemically induced tumours did have distinctly different immunogenic properties brought about the re-emergence of interest in this subject. This is well illustrated by the increase in publications on tumour immunology during the past few years (Morton, 1974) (Fig. 10.1). The use of such syngenetic animal strains and transplanted tumours has not answered all the questions and the field is once again developing along the lines of the early explorers in tumour immunology, but with the benefit of the meth-

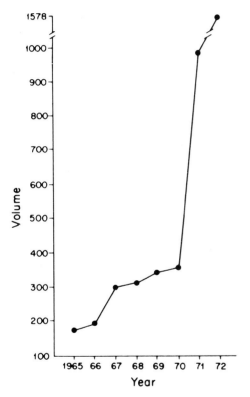

Fig. 10.1 Showing the increase in publications on the subject of tumour immunology since 1965. (*From* Morton, 1974)

odologies and techniques worked out in these animal models.

Perhaps one of the greatest dangers of a syngeneic animal system with transplantable tumours is on the one hand the complete removal of the individuality of the immune response, which in patients with cancer may be more important than we realise, and secondly the fact that the long latent period of develop-

ment of the tumour is not seen and, therefore, the immunological challenge to the host may well be different. For instance, the timing of immune reactions following antigen stimulation is not appreciably different in the mouse and man, yet few murine tumours persist for months and certainly not for years. It is not sufficient, therefore, to relate the life-span of such species to the duration of tumour progression in immunological terms. Evidence will now be reviewed for the presence of immune reactivity in patients with malignant melanoma as an example, and the mechanisms for failure of this immune control will be discussed in detail.

EVIDENCE OF IMMUNE REACTIONS IN MELANOMA FROM CLINICAL OBSERVATIONS

Several observers have noted over the years some of the variation in the duration of the different stages of development in patients with melanoma (Fig. 10.2), and the variation in the natural history of this tumour and many other human cancers have been well known to clinicians for many years (Coley and Hoguet, 1916). Almost certainly, the most striking phenomenon in this respect is spontaneous regression. This controversial subject has been explored by a number of people over the years, and in patients with malignant melanoma this has been clearly recorded from a number of different centres. Everson and Cole (1966) in a classical monograph reported several examples of spontaneous regression in a collected series, and more recently McGovern (1975) has presented a detailed analysis of the phenomena, pointing out the very important subvariety in which partial regression of tumours, particularly in melanoma, may occur with more frequency than the more dramatic complete spontaneous regression.

A rather unique form of spontaneous regression can be seen in melanomas presenting as lymph node metastases with no obvious primary (Fig. 10.3). This was first described in 1896 by Eberman of Petrograd and various

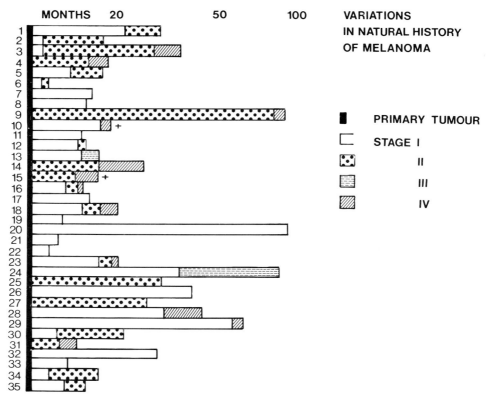

Fig. 10.2   A schematic representation of the variations in progression of melanoma stage by stage. The stages of melanoma referred to in the text and in this figure are: Stage 1—Primary malignant melanoma (any level of invasion). Stage 2—Regional lymph node involvement with or without recurrence or satellites in the draining area of the primary tumour. Stage 3—Disease extending beyond the regional lymph nodes but not including parenchymal organ involvement (skin metastasis only). Stage 4—Widespread dissemination including viscera.

reports have been added to the literature since. In some instances including the author's own experience, spontaneous regression of the primary tumours is perhaps the best explanation. As Kopf (1971) has pointed out, although melanoma represents only between 1 and 3 per cent of all cancers, it accounts for 15 per cent of cases of well-documented spontaneous regression.

Bodenham (1968), in his extensive study of over more than 20 years of malignant melanoma, emphasised the way in which even established metastatic disease may alter. He showed on several occasions the phenomenon of so-called smouldering disease, in which nodules appear and disappear on the same leg

over a period of months or years (Fig. 10.4). Delay of metastases is another manifestation suggestive of a host defence mechanism, and the best example undoubtedly would be the appearance of metastases in the liver, sometimes many years after removal of the eye in intra-ocular malignant melanoma. Since the eye has no lymphatic drainage, the tumour of necessity must have already metastasised prior to the enucleation, and yet a long period of time may elapse before these metastases appear clinically in the liver. This cannot simply be explained away on the basis of a slowness of growth of these tumours, since the speed with which this tumour may progress after clinical detection varies considerably. Further evi-

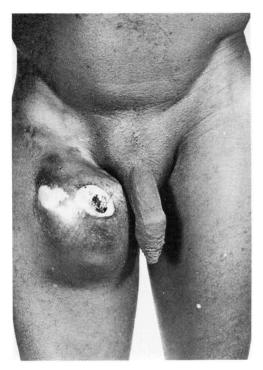

Fig. 10.3 Malignant melanoma presenting as a lymph node metastasis, with no detectable primary tumour. (*From* Lewis, 1971)

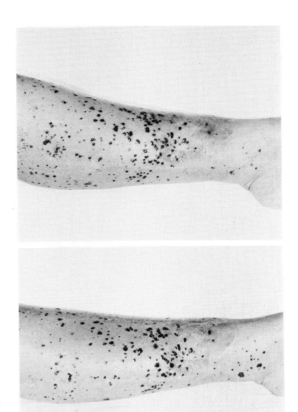

Fig. 10.4 An example of secondary malignant melanoma on the leg of a patient showing changes over a period of time with lesions disappearing and new lesions arising. (*From* Bodenham, 1968)

dence for the possibility of immunologically determined host factors resulted from studies on the so-called halo naevus phenomenon in which a pigmented mole develops a halo of depigmentation and subsequently disappears (Sutton, 1916) (Fig. 10.5). In some of the clinical cases of malignant melanoma depigmented halos may also occur around them, and as will be seen later, similar immunological factors may be involved.

Studies in Africa, where melanomas occur predominantly on soles of the feet, resulted in a much clearer picture in terms of host–tumour relationships. Three groups of patients were easily identifiable since the primary lesions were in the same anatomical site and the position of the regional lymph nodes were identical in all cases (Lewis, 1967a). Patients with melanoma were classified as group 1 where the tumour remained localised for months or years, group 2 where the tumour grew rapidly in a matter of weeks and group 3 where the primary tumour had regressed or was regressing leaving regional metastases. Studies including pathology of the tumour, the sex-ratios, tribal factors, age and other criteria showed no differences between the groups, and it was concluded that some factor, possibly in the serum, prevented the one group of tumours from metastasising until late (Lewis and Kiryabwire, 1968). It was these observations that led to an exploration for serum factors as a means of explaining why tumour growth locally did not produce blood-borne metastases until late in the disease (Lewis, 1967b). A

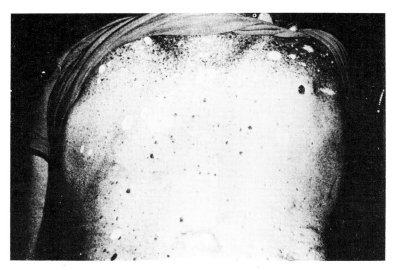

Fig. 10.5   A patient with multiple halo naevi and widespread cutaneous secondary malignant melanoma. (Reproduced by kind permission of Dr W. H. Clark, Jr)

selection of the main references to clinical evidence for host reactivity in melanoma is shown in Table 10.1.

EVIDENCE FOR IMMUNE REACTIVITY DERIVED FROM PATHOLOGICAL OBSERVATIONS

This can be seen in the various cellular infiltrates which occur particularly in primary tumours. This subject has been extensively reviewed by Underwood (1974) who quotes Wade in 1908 '... the tumour is borne away on a tide of lymphocytes'. The great pathologist Virchow was certainly aware of the presence of lymphocytes in tumours and even suggested that this implied an origin of such tumours in chronic inflammation (Virchow, 1863). Again, melanoma is a useful tumour in this respect since it is possible to diagnose the disease at a very early stage and follow the various relationships between cell infiltrates and progression of tumour. It was noted very early on that lymphocytes in many instances invade the primary tumours (Handley, 1907) and also that melanin-containing macrophages were often seen in large numbers. A recent re-emer-gence of interest by immunologists in the macrophage–tumour cell interaction has occurred (Evans and Alexander, 1972; Hibbs, Lambert and Remington, 1972), although these events were well documented by the early pathologists and even earlier by Metchnikoff and his colleagues in elegant studies on the phagocytic functions of these cells (Himmelweitt, 1957). Several others have shown tumour cell phagocytosis *in vitro* and in addition *in vivo* (The *et al.*, 1972; LeJeune, 1973). One of the major difficulties in correlating the degree of lymphocytic infiltrate or plasma cell infiltrate in tumours has been the variable stage in which these tumours are removed. Certainly in the African series where enormous tumours were present with surface ulceration it was difficult to ensure that these cells were reacting to tumour rather than to infection and other factors. Little (1972), however, and Thompson (1972) have clearly shown that lymphocytic infiltration and plasma cell infiltrates can be correlated with some degree of prognosis and of considerable interest is the disappearance both morphologically and functionally of lymphocytes and monocytes as the tumours progress from level III and level IV and beyond (Roubin *et al.*, 1975; Bailly, 1972).

Table 10.1   Evidence of host antitumour reactivity in human melanoma

Handley	1907	Observation on natural history. Lymphocytes in tumour cells by histo-pathology
Sumner and Foraker	1960	
Everson and Cole	1966	Spontaneous regression of metastatic malignant melanoma
Todd *et al.*	1966	
Eberman	1896	
Coley and Hoguet	1916	
Pack and Miller	1961	
Das Gupta *et al.*	1963	Presumptive regression of 1° melanoma with persisting lymph node
Smith and Stehlin	1965	metastases (so-called occult 1° melanoma)
McGovern	1966	
Milton *et al.*	1967	
Lewis	1967a	
Petersen *et al.*	1962	
McGovern	1972	
Little	1972	Partial regression of primary cutaneous melanoma
McGovern	1975	
Wilbur and Hartmann	1931	
Allen and Spitz	1953	
MacDonald	1963	Variations in delay of metastatic spread without therapeutic inter-ference apart from surgery
Bodenham	1968	
Lewis and Kiryabwire	1968	

Although there have been recent suggestions that lymphocytes may in fact cause tumour progression in some instances (Prehn, 1972), the data from human melanoma would suggest that they can be related to early successful reaction with the tumour.

Inflammation surrounding a tumour not only is a clinical hallmark of malignant melanoma but also is typical of the early stage of involution of the supposedly benign naevus that develops a halo of depigmentation and is referred to as leukoderma acquisitum centrifugum, Sutton's naevus or the halo naevus (Findlay, 1957; Kopf, Morrill and Silberberg, 1965; Césarini, Bonneau and Calas, 1968; Ebner and Neibauer, 1968; Stegmaier, Becker and Medenica, 1969; Wayte and Helwig, 1968; Epstein *et al.*, 1973; Gauthier *et al.*, 1975). This is a clinicopathological phenomenon of great interest since it is clear evidence for auto-destruction of a melanotic tumour. Why a benign mole should after many years develop redness and inflammation and eventually regress is a question that requires explanation,

since there is evidence connecting this lesion with malignant melanoma. It is clear that the halo naevus and early malignant melanoma have several features in common, such as the presence of an infiltrate and antibodies in the circulation of patients that are reactive with cytoplasmic antigens of melanoma cells (Copeman *et al.*, 1973). Indeed, the histological appearances of early inflamed halo naevus before development of the associated halo of depigmentation may easily be mistaken for early malignant melanoma (McGovern, 1975). These immunological and morphological associations led to the suggestion that the halo naevus represents a seldom seen interim stage in the normal successful rejection of a developing malignant melanoma (Lewis and Copeman, 1972).

Recently, Jacobs *et al.*, (1975) and Rowden and Lewis (1975a) have reported studies of a number of cases of early halo naevus. A significant observation in both studies was the finding of close apposition or peripolesis of mononuclear cells with naevus cells.

Cell-to-cell contact appeared to be an attendant feature of the extensive vacuolar degeneration of naevus cells that was seen (Fig. 10.6). The exact nature of the cytotoxic event which seems to result from the close apposition of lymphoid cells to tumour cell membranes is not known.

The destruction of the epidermal melanocytes in the immediate vicinity of the regressing naevus may be produced by similar cell contacts. However, these contacts are not as frequent as in the naevus area, and it may be that the vacuolar degeneration results from diffusible cytotoxic substances such as lympho-

toxin produced by the lymphocytes (Fig. 10.7).

Recent ultrastructural investigations of early superficial spreading melanomas (Roubin et al., 1975) have demonstrated the presence of mononuclear cells forming close apposition to tumour cells, similar to those reported above. Generally, however, there was little evidence of successful cell destruction, although this was mentioned as an occasional observation. Studies in our laboratory of lymph nodes with varying degrees of metastatic melanoma involvement have shown that similar interactions

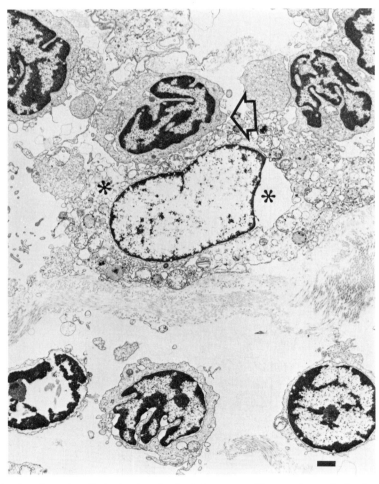

Fig. 10.6   Infiltrating lymphocytic cells in the dermis of a halo naevus. Mononuclear cells in close association with a naevus cell (*arrow*). Severe vacuolar degeneration of a naevus cell(*).   ×7500 (marker = 1 micron)

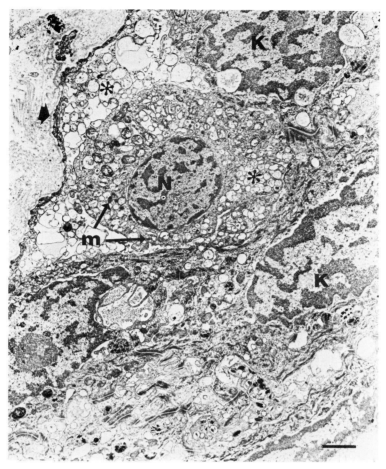

Fig. 10.7 Vacuolar degeneration of a melanocyte in the epidermis of a halo naevus specimen. There is intracellular and intercellular vacuolation (*). No evidence for apposition of lymphoid cells. K=keratinocyte nucleus; M=melanin granules; N=nucleus of malanocyte. Basal lamina indicated by the arrow. × 13 500 (marker=1 micron)

occur between host cells and tumour cells. In partially involved nodes, these cell-to-cell contacts are capable of producing destruction of tumour cells, once again with the morphological appearance of vacuolar degeneration (Fig. 10.8).

The fact that Underwood and Carr (1972) in their detailed analysis of densely infiltrated tumours failed to demonstrate that the close apposition of host cells to tumour cells resulted in any destructive event likely to limit tumour growth indicates that there is probably some

mechanism operating whereby the host cells are prevented from expressing their full cytotoxic capacities in established tumours. Consideration of these possible blocking factors is dealt with elsewhere in this review. Clearly, further study of the halo naevus will be of great value since it provides an opportunity to establish in the human the possible mechanisms of host cell destruction of neoplastic melanocytes.

The presence of plasma cells in early melanomas according to Little (1972) may, however, have quite a different relationship

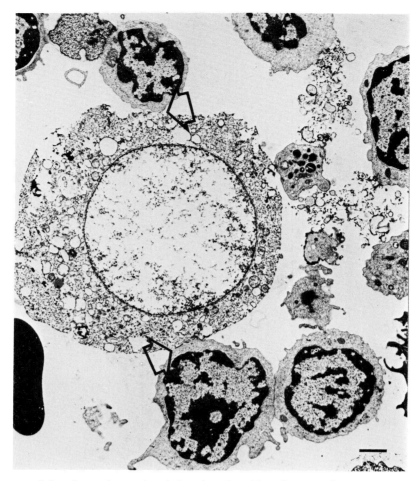

Fig. 10.8   Tumour cell–lymphocyte interactions in lymph nodes with malignant melanoma involvement. Cells stained to show surface immunoglobulin with anti-γ-peroxidase γ-negative cells in close contact with a degenerating tumour cell (*arrows*). Vacuolar degeneration present in the tumour cell. $\times 10\,200$ (marker = 1 micron)

and be a poor prognostic factor. The implications and reasons for this will be discussed subsequently. The key references to this aspect of the subject are summarised in Table 10.2.

In summary, therefore, at this point it can be stated that the natural history of malignant melanoma and its histopathology strongly suggests that the host can react in some way against the tumour with variable degrees of success. The tumour, although amenable to diagnosis at an early stage, can in fact produce metastases via the lymphatics and the bloodstream and involve extremely widespread organ systems. Despite this, the time intervals between these stages may vary considerably. These factors all led to the questions of whether these host reactions could be shown to be of an immunological nature.

In the following section, discussion will focus on the methods for detecting specific and non-specific immune reactivity in such patients.

Table 10.2   Evidence for host–tumour interactions from morphological studies

Handley	1907	
Couperus and Rucker	1954	
Williams *et al.*	1968	
Cochran	1969	
Thompson	1972	Histological and in some studies electron microscopical observations on host cell infiltrates in tumours and correlation with prognosis
Little	1972	
Burg and Braun-Falco	1972	
McLeod	1972	
McGovern	1975	
Roubin *et al.*	1975	
Iversen *et al.*	1976	
Lieberman *et al.*	1974	Histopathological changes in nodules after BCG treatment correlated with cell-mediated immunity
Lieberman *et al.*	1975	
Humble *et al.*	1956	Composition of host cells within tumours or in peripheral blood. Monocyte–lymphocytes in primary tissue culture of tumours—emperipolesis
The *et al.*	1972	*In vivo* phagocytosis of melanoma cells
Lejeune	1973	Macrophages in melanoma
Nind *et al.*	1973	T and B cell content of intratumour lymphocytes
Hersh *et al.*	1975	Lymphocyte–monocyte counts in melanoma
Gauci	1975	Macrophage content of melanomas
Bourgoin *et al.*	1975	T cell levels in malignant melanoma patients' blood related to stage of disease
Claudy *et al.*	1975	Significant drop in active E rosettes in rapidly growing melanoma
Lewis, Proctor, Thomson *et al.*	1976	Immunoglobulin-positive lymphoid cells in melanoma

IDENTIFICATION OF TUMOUR ANTIGENS

There are two basic approaches to the identification of antigens in tumours. In the first instance, the tumour cells may be disrupted and various subfractions obtained. These can then be tested for antigenicity by immunising other species such as rabbits, goats, etc. and testing the reaction of such antisera against the fractions or whole tumour cells observed; alternatively, the subcellular fractions may be utilised for skin testing in the individual or against immune components of that individual, such as lymphocytes and antibody.

The second approach is the reverse of the above, in that initially it is necessary to demonstrate that the individual can mount an immune response, either humoral or cell mediated, against his own tumour or against the tumours of other individuals, and then to further show that these immune responses are qualitatively different against the tumour, compared to normal cells from that individual. The latter method then allows one to identify which of the various tumour products or components is immunogenic to the host. Both these approaches have been used and reported extensively and will now be considered in more detail.

Since the early part of this century when Von Dungen used emulsified tumour preparations and showed that injection into the skin caused reddening and swelling (Currie, 1972), numerous investigators have used this approach to demonstrate that tumour antigens may elicit a response which appears to be specific (Stewart, 1969). The specificity, however, varied with the different investigations. In addition, extracts of tumour cells, particularly melanoma, have been shown to cause skin test reactivity and also in some instances a blastogenic response from the patients' peripheral blood lymphocytes.

Fluid obtained from an individual patient with a cystic degenerate melanoma was shown to elicit both skin test reactivity in one series (Jehn, Nathanson and Schwartz, 1970) and also reactivity measured by the migration inhibition technique by another group (Cochran, Jehn and Gothoska, 1972). More recently, reports have shown that relatively specific components of melanoma cell membranes can produce such reactivity in individual patients and a combined study from the U.S.S.R. and the U.S.A. showed that the same glycolipoprotein produced identical reactions in patients from both those countries, indicating even higher degrees of tumour specificity (Gorodilova and Hollinshead, 1975). The major reports using this approach are summarised in Table 10.3.

On several occasions melanoma extracts of varying compositions have been injected into rabbits (Goodwin et al., 1972), goats (Ghose et al., 1972) and more recently into chimpan-zees (Metzgar et al., 1973). The sera after absorption with normal human tissues and serum have also been used in the treatment of melanoma patients, in some instances by coupling the antisera to chemotherapeutic agents. Here the authors claimed that some tumour nodules disappeared during this therapy (Ghose et al., 1975).

DEMONSTRATION OF SPONTANEOUS IMMUNE REACTIVITY OF INDIVIDUALS AGAINST MELANOMA

Humoral immunity

There are numerous methods for detecting the presence of circulating antibodies in the sera of patients with malignancy (Lewis, 1972). The presence of antibody directed against melanoma cells or antigens has been one of the most extensive areas of investigation and was originally carried out in an attempt to explain why the local tumour continues to grow and yet blood borne metastases appeared late in the disease (or not at all). These antibodies were demonstrated by means of complement-dependent cytotoxicity (Pulvertaft, 1959), against live tumour target cells (Lewis, 1967b; Bodurtha et al., 1975) (Fig. 10.9), and also by means of immunofluorescence both against the surface of live tumour cells (Klein et al., 1966) and against cytoplasmic contents in snap-frozen (Nairn, 1969) or fixed cell preparations (Morton et al., 1968) (Fig. 10.10). The immunofluorescence technique first developed by Coons, Creech and Jones (1941), has been

Table 10.3   *In vivo* immune responses to melanoma

Hughes and Lytton	1964	
Katz and Digby	1965	
Stewart	1969	
Fass et al.	1970	
Blumming et al.	1972	
Mavligit et al.	1973a	Effects of tumour cells or extracts by skin testing
Hollinshead et al.	1974	
Char et al.	1974	
Gorodilova and Hollinshead	1975	
Hollinshead	1975	

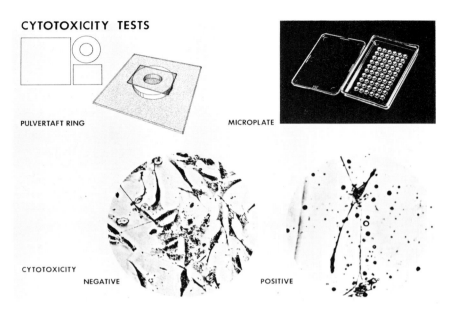

Fig. 10.9   Some examples of complement-dependent cytotoxicity tests. (*From* Lewis, 1973a, with permission of J. B. Lippincott Co.)

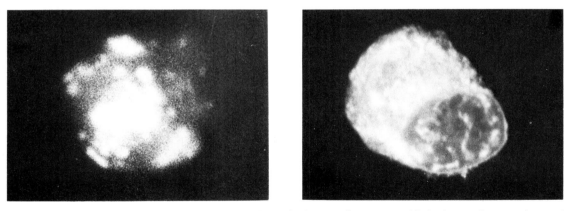

Fig. 10.10   Melanoma cells with antibody reactions shown by immunofluorescence. (a) Against surface membrane of cell. (b) In the cytoplasm of cell.

used widely in biological studies, but the need for very careful controls and standardisation must be emphasised (Lewis, 1974a). One of the major problems in assessing antitumour antibodies has been a lack of methods for quantitation, apart from procedures such as fluorescent index or percentage of staining cells (Phillips and Lewis, 1970).

The complement-dependent cytotoxic assay has been modified to include some degree of quantitation (Bodurtha *et al.*, 1975). Methods of quantitation of fluorescent antibodies techniques have been described on several occasions (Goldman, 1960, 1967) and the subject has been extensively reviewed (Goldman, 1968; Nairn, 1969; Holborow, 1970; Ploem,

1970). In most instances, this involved the use of microfluorimetry and required complicated and expensive equipment. In more recent times simpler modifications have been described, including a comparator microscope system using a slit-lamp comparator built into the eyepiece. This allows a semiquantitative assessment of the degree of intensity of fluorescence (Haskill and Raymond, 1973). This method has been used in scanning antibody responses in melanoma patients, particularly against cytoplasmic antigen in smear preparations (Lewis and Raymond, 1975). Antibodies directed against surface membrane of melanoma cells have also been detected and quantitation estimates performed using a more sophisticated microscope with microfluorimetry. This allows the intensity of fluorescence to be measured on the surface of individual melanoma cells (Lewis, Avis, Phillips *et al.*, 1973) (Figs. 10.11 and 10.12). In addition, antibody has been identified using methods such as immunodiffusion against melanoma extracts and by immuno-electrophoresis and

passive haemagglutination. Table 10.4 summarises additional references from the literature on antimelanoma antibodies.

Cell-mediated immunity

Skin testing. Investigators have used most of the standard available methods for assessing cell-mediated immunity in malignant melanoma including the skin testing already partly described, in which either tumour antigen or non-related antigens are injected into the skin and cutaneous delayed hypersensitivity reactions are noted and measured. The major problem with this method is the difficulty of assessing the degree of response and often the specificity; but now with more refined preparation, claims are being made for increased specificity and better quantitation.

Lymphocyte blastogenic response. The response of peripheral blood lymphocytes to tumour antigen preparations, either crude extracts or more refined subcellular fractions, is another method which has been used exten-

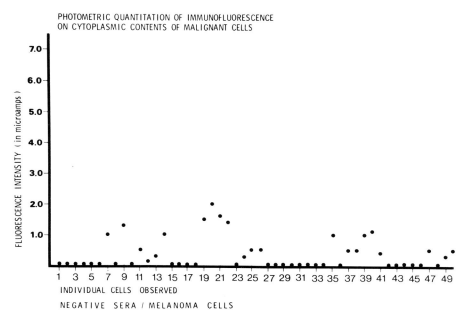

Fig. 10.11   Quantitation of immunofluorescent reaction on surface of melanoma cells measured by microfluorimetry. (*From* Lewis, Avis, Phillips *et al.*, 1973)

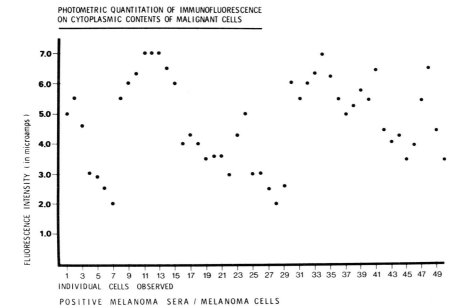

Fig. 10.12   Quantitation of immunofluorescent reaction on surface of melanoma cells measured by microfluorimetry. (*From* Lewis, Avis, Phillips *et al.*, 1973)

Table 10.4   Evidence for humoral immunity in melanoma

		Cytotoxicity of serum antibodies
Lewis	1967b	Individual specificity and related to stages of disease (fresh tumour cells)
Lewis *et al.*	1969	
Gray *et al.*	1971	
Nairn *et al.*	1972	Some individual specificity—not related to stage of disease (fresh tumour cells)
Della Porta *et al.*	1973	Fresh tumour cells
Bodurtha *et al.*	1975	Fresh tumour cells—individual specificity
Canevari *et al.*	1975	Melanoma cell lines—not individually specific
		Immuno-fluorescence detection of serum tumour level or tumour-bound immunoglobulin
Oettgen *et al.*	1968	Anticytoplasmic IF against established melanoma cell line
Morton *et al.*	1968	Anticytoplasmic IF in fresh tumour preparation
Lewis *et al.*	1969	Anticytoplasmic IF and antimembrane IF correlation between antimembrane and cytotoxicity
Muna *et al.*	1969	Cytoplasmic IF 100% cross reacting. No membrane IF seen in 5/5 cases
Romsdahl and Cox	1970	Membrane and cytoplasmic IF with higher rate of cross reactivity
Phillips and Lewis	1970	Cytoplasmic IF specificity and degree of cross reactivity
Morton *et al.*	1970	Membrane immunofluorescence and cytoplasmic. 29% of normal blood donors gave positive tests
Phillips	1971	Improvement in method of immunofluorescence decrease in non-specific reactions
Lewis, Phillips, Cook *et al.*	1971	Blocking of individually specific antimembrane antibody by autologous negative serum—suggestive of anti-idiotypic antibody

(*continued*)

Table 10.4 (*continued*)

Morton *et al.*	1971	Antimembrane and anticytoplasmic IF with evidence that autologous reactions tend to be greater than allogeneic
Rahi	1971	Antibodies for IF against ocular melanoma
Lewis and Phillips	1972a	Individual specificity of antimembrane antibodies. Cross-absorption with allogeneic cells
McBride *et al.*	1972	Antinuclear and nuclear IF seen most frequently
Nairn *et al.*	1972	Membrane and cytoplasm IF. No clear stage relationship
Lewis and Phillips	1972b	Separation of two distinct antibodies against membrane and cytoplasm in individual sera
Lewis, Avis, Phillips *et al.*.	1973	Differences in time relationship between various antibody–antigen reactions
Whitehouse	1973	Auto-antibodies reactive in melanoma
Federman *et al.*	1974a	Antimembrane and anticytoplasmic antibodies in ocular melanoma
Federman *et al.*	1974b	Negative reactivity of anti-ocular melanoma sera against normal choroidal melanocytes
Hartmann *et al.*	1974	Antitumour antibodies and anti-IgG anti-antibodies
O'Neill and Romsdahl	1974	IgG antibodies as blocking antibodies in malignant melanoma
Wood and Barth	1974	Methods of fixation for cytoplasmic IF in melanoma cell lines and fresh cells
Gupta and Morton	1975	Tumour-bound antibody detected by complement fixation
Macher *et al.*	1975	Cross-reacting antibodies against melanoma cell line membranes
The *et al.*	1975	Antimembrane immunofluorescence against melanoma cell lines
Lewis, Proctor, Thomson *et al.*	1976	Antimembrane antibodies not detectable in high levels on solid tumour deposits *in vivo*
Lewis, Hartmann and Jerry	1976	Anticytoplasmic antibodies related to the presence of anti-IgG antibodies

Miscellaneous methods
Immunodiffusion, immunoelectrophoresis, immune adherence

McKenna *et al.*	1964	Immunodiffusion
Czajowski *et al.*	1967	Gel diffusion against tumour extracts
Lewis, Phillips, Cook *et al.*	1971	Haemagglutination, immunodiffusion and immunoelectrophoresis
Lewis and Phillips	1972	Affinity chromatography of antibodies on antigen columns
Carrel and Theilkaes	1973	Double diffusion—antigen in urine
Gupta and Morton	1975	Complement fixation
Macher *et al.*	1975	Immune adherence with formalin fixed melanoma cells on red cells
DeVries *et al.*	1975	Immune adherence for the presence of complement fixed antibody against cell lines (no correlation with stage of disease)

Xenogenic antimelanoma antibody production

Viza and Phillips	1971	Rabbit antisera
Goodwin *et al.*	1972	Rabbit antisera
Ghose *et al.*	1972	Goat antisera
Metzgar *et al.*	1973	Monkey antisera
Stuhlmiller and Seigler	1975	Chimpanzee antisera
Viza *et al.*	1975	Rabbit antisera

sively. The blastogenic response of these lymphocytes (Stjernswärd *et al.*, 1968) has been measured by various procedures, including uptake of radioisotope by the dividing cells or based on morphological studies (Cooper, 1970; Kanner, Mardiney and Mairgi, 1970).

Leucocyte adherence inhibition. More recently a method described as the leucocyte adherence inhibition assay has been described by Halliday and his colleagues in Australia (Halliday and Miller, 1972) and it has been used by several other investigators particularly in studies on melanoma. Here the principle is to show that an antigen can cause buffy coat leucocytes to become non-adherent to glass and further to demonstrate that this is specific for the antigen concerned and occurs only at reasonable levels in individuals who have recent or continued exposure to this particular tumour. The leucocyte adherence inhibition test with some recent modification (mentioned later) is diagrammatically represented in Figure 10.13.

appeared in recent years using this assay. There has been conflict in the results, some people claiming that it is not tumour specific (Takasugi, Mickey and Teraski, 1974), whereas others have shown that it can distinguish the tumour patient from the normal population (O'Toole et al., 1972 and 1974). We have recently used this particular test extensively and by carrying out appropriate normal controls, were able to distinguish a population of melanoma patients, particularly those in the early stages of disease from the normal population. In addition, we were able to show changes of reactivity following immune manipulation (Roy et al., 1976).

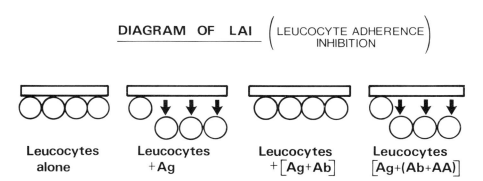

Fig. 10.13 Diagrammatic representation of the leucocyte adherence inhibition test. Showing adherence of buffy coat leucocytes to haemocytometer counting chambers, and subsequent non-adherence when mixed with specific tumour antigen. The effect of interference with this system using serum containing tumour antibody and anti-antibody is represented. Ag—tumour antigen; Ab—antitumour antibody; AA—anti-antibody. (*From* Lewis et al., 1976b)

Lymphocytotoxicity

This is perhaps one of the most widely studied tests for cell-mediated immunity (Takasugi and Klein, 1970; Takasugi, Mickey and Takasugi, 1973; Hellström, Hellström, Sjögren et al., 1971) and it measures the cytotoxic ability of peripheral blood lymphocytes, usually purified in some way such as layering on Ficoll isopaque, to separate lymphocytes from other components of the blood. These cells are then applied to monolayers of tumour cells. A number of extensive reports have

The colony inhibition assay

The colony inhibition assay described by Hellström (1967) is a method for showing the effect that populations of lymphocytes may have on the ability of tumour cells to grow in colonies (Fig. 10.14). Thus, although it does not produce lysis of the tumour cell, it prevents growth. Numerous investigators have demonstrated that this perhaps is the one test with the most difficulty in reproduction. However, it has now been well established by groups other than the original authors (Baldwin et al.,

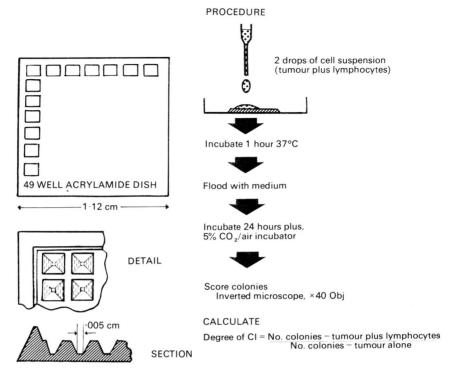

PROCEDURE

2 drops of cell suspension
(tumour plus lymphocytes)

Incubate 1 hour 37°C

Flood with medium

Incubate 24 hours plus,
5% CO_2/air incubator

Score colonies
Inverted microscope, ×40 Obj

CALCULATE

$$\text{Degree of CI} = \frac{\text{No. colonies} - \text{tumour plus lymphocytes}}{\text{No. colonies} - \text{tumour alone}}$$

49 WELL ACRYLAMIDE DISH

◄——— 1·12 cm ———►

DETAIL

·005 cm

SECTION

Fig. 10.14   Diagrammatic summary of principle of colony inhibition of tumour cells by patient's lymphocytes or serum. (*Adapted from* Haskill, 1973)

1974a; Heppner *et al.*, 1973) and can be a very effective procedure.

Antibody-dependent cell-mediated immunity

In this procedure, the addition of antibody provides the specificity which allows cell-mediated immunity to become effective on a non-specific basis (Hersey, MacLennon and Campbell, 1973; MacLennon and Harding, 1973). The test has not been used extensively in human melanomas but certainly has been shown to be a useful assay under many other circumstances (Landazuri, Kedar and Fahey, 1975).

Leucocyte migration inhibition (LMI)

LMI tests have also been used widely in human tumour immunology and in particular

with respect to melanoma; several authors (Cochran, Spilg, Mackie *et al.*, 1972) have shown that this is a useful means of demonstrating a specific reaction in individual patients against tumours. In this respect it has been shown that the tumour extract is able to inhibit migration of leucocytes from capillary tubes, and factors have been identified called migration inhibition factors (MIF) in these circumstances.

Tests of macrophage function in malignancy

The role of macrophages is now becoming more established in tumour immunology. In fact macrophages were recognised by the early pathologists as being an important component of melanoma. More recently there have been assays to measure the effect of macrophages either by inhibition of migration or chemotaxic experiments. In addition, the ability of these cells under various circumstances to carry out phagocytosis has been the subject of much study (Lejeune, 1975). In a study by The *et al.* (1972), material was examined from 37 melanoma patients in which four of these had some degree of tumour cell phagocytosis. Antibody eluted from tumour cells in lymph node metastases was shown to induce phagocytosis of cultured melanoma cells.

These observations are similar to that described by Evans and Alexander of their specific macrophage 'arming factor' in experimental tumour systems (1972). Some of the key reports from the literature regarding the identification of cell-mediated immunity in melanoma are summarised in Table 10.5.

Table 10.5 Evidence for *in vitro* cell-mediated immunity in patients with melanoma

		Blastogenic response of lymphoid cells in tumours
Savel	1969	Reaction in one case during spontaneous regression
Nagel	1970	Cross-reactivity between twins: related to stage of disease
Cooper	1970	Stimulation of lymphocytes by melanoma
Jehn *et al.*	1970	Cross-reactivity between melanoma patients against a single melanoma extract
Mavligit *et al.*	1973b	Cross-reactivity between melanoma patients demonstrated
Ambus *et al.*	1974	Clinical stage correlation demonstrated
Butterworth *et al.*	1974	Mixed lymphocyte reaction. Reactivity correlates with stage of disease. More clearly demonstrated in early stages
Hersh *et al.*	1975	Blastogenic responses of lymphocytes related to other immune parameters
DeGast *et al.*	1975	Alterations in patient lymphocyte response in PHA and non-tumour antigens less often seen in rapidly advancing tumours
		Anti-tumour effects of lymphocytes on target tumour cells (cytotoxicity and/or colony inhibition)
Hellström	1967	Colony inhibition
Hellström, Hellström, *et al.*	1971	Cytotoxicity (allogeneic)
Fossati *et al.*	1971	Cytotoxicity (allogeneic), also humoral immune reactions
Currie *et al.*	1971	Cytotoxicity (autologous)
Nairn *et al.*	1972	Modification of Pulvertaft ring test with lymphocyte (autologous). No clinical correlation
Currie and Basham	1972	Microtoxicity
DeVries *et al.*	1972	Allogeneic
Nind *et al.*	1973	Cytotoxicity of peripheral blood and lymph node lymphocytes
Heppner *et al.*	1973	Colony inhibition, microtoxicity and serum blocking tested sequentially
Hellström, Warner *et al.*	1973	Colony inhibition, cytotoxicity and serum blocking
Hellström, Hellström *et al.*	1973	Normal blood donor lymphocytes cytotoxicity of melanoma cells
Byrne *et al.*	1973	Colony inhibition and microtoxicity
Mukherji *et al.*	1973	Lymphocytotoxicity and antibody studies related to stage of disease
Pihl *et al.*	1974	Electron microscopical study of lymphocytotoxicity
Roenigk *et al.*	1975	Lymphocytotoxicity and serum blocking against melanoma and halo naevi
Heppner *et al.*	1975	Problems with microcytotoxicity as an assay
Hersey	1975	Explanations for some degree of non-specificity in the method of microcytotoxicity
Hersh *et al.*	1975	Microcytotoxicity measured by titrated proline in conjunction with melanoma cell line
DeVries *et al.*	1975	Microcytotoxicity, T and non-T cell populations compared
Embleton and Price	1975	Microcytotoxicity and inhibition by melanoma membrane extracts

(continued)

Table 10.5 (*continued*)

Pavie-Fischer *et al.*	1975	Lymphocytotoxicity measured by chromium .51 release
Peter *et al.*	1975	
Riethmüller *et al.*	1975	Lymphocytotoxicity measured by H³ proline release
Pilch *et al.*	1975	Lymphocytotoxicity of normal lymphocytes treated with immune RNA from 'cured' melanoma patient

Leucocyte migration inhibition (LMI)

Cochran, Jehn and Gothoska	1972	LMI assay related to stage of disease
Cochran, Spilg *et al.*	1972	Postoperative depression of cell-mediated immunity
Segall *et al.*	1972	Sequential studies in patients undergoing immunotherapy
Falk *et al.*	1973	
Cochran, Mackie *et al.*	1973	Technical problems of LMI—solved by use of formalin fixed cells
Cochran, Thomas *et al.*	1973	Modification by surgical treatment of patients
Cochran *et al.*	1975	Correlation between skin testing and LMI with melanoma extracts
Herberman *et al.*	1975	

Leucocyte adherence inhibition (LAI)

Halliday and Miller	1972	Description of LAI test
Maluish and Halliday	1974	Blocking of LAI with serum factors
Halliday *et al.*	1974	
Hartmann *et al.*	1974	Interaction between antimelanoma cytoplasmic antibody and anti (Fab¹)₂ Anti-antibodies using LAI test
Grosser and Thompson	1975	Modification of LAI test using a tube method

Antibody dependent cell-mediated lysis of target cells

| Peter *et al.* | 1975 | |
| Hersey *et al.* | 1973 | |

MELANOMA ANTIGENS AND THEIR SPECIFICITY

A major area of controversy in the field of tumour immunology is the question of specificity of tumour antigens. Here terms such as tumour specific transplantation antigen (TSTA), tumour associated antigen (TAA), tumour specific antigens (TSA) and even carcino-embryonic antigens (CEA) are used extensively. The concept that a tumour antigen must be a new antigen and, therefore, can only occur on the tumour cell and not on normal cells has been perhaps one of the major dogmas in tumour immunology. This limited concept of tumour antigens is now coming under critical review, in that the possibility exists that tumour antigens may be abnormal expressions of normal tissue antigens. A number of observers have shown the presence of auto-

antibodies against other tissue components in malignancy and related these to certain tumour tissues (Whitehouse and Holborow, 1971). Whatever the ultimate nature of the tumour antigens turns out to be, some evidence has been put forward illustrating that a quantitative difference exists between the antigens on the tumour and on the normal tissues. This has been demonstrated indirectly by absorption procedures where a variety of tissues or unrelated tumours fail to absorb out the antibody in comparison with the fresh tumour extract (Lewis, Ikonopisov *et al.*, 1969).

Another approach has been to show that an antibody reacting with tumour cells shows low or no reactivity with normal cells using the same methodology. In some instances investigators have used tissue culture cells, fibroblasts or fetal cells and some have used or attempted to use the cell of origin of the tumours. In a

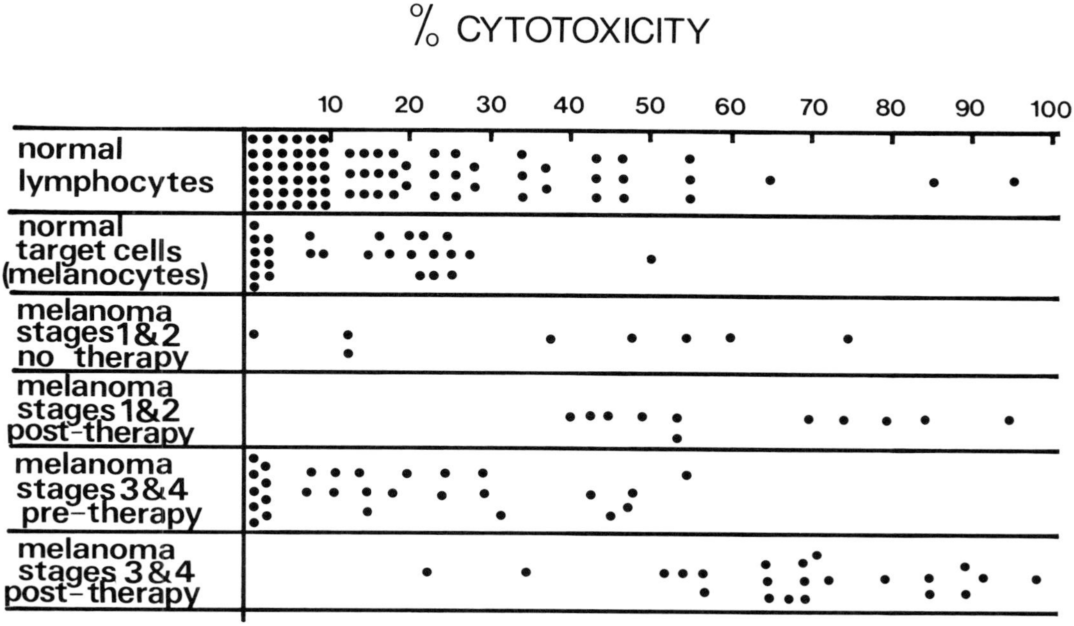

Fig. 10.15   The degree of cytotoxicity of autologous lymphocytes and normal lymphocytes against melanoma cells.

study of ocular melanoma, for instance, it was clearly demonstrated that antibody could react against the ocular melanoma cells but not against choroidal melanocytes obtained from either the same eye or from normal eyes (Federman *et al.*, 1974; Federman, J. L., Lewis, M. G. and Clarke, W. H., 1974). Similar lack of cytotoxicity with lymphocytes against tumour cells and choroidal melanocytes or fibroblasts has been demonstrated (Roy *et al.*, 1976) (Fig. 10.15). Differences in reactivity between extracts of tumour cells and extracts of normal cells, both in the LAI test and in skin testing, have been repeatedly demonstrated (Maluish and Halliday, 1974; Hollinshead, 1975; Grosser and Thompson, 1974). There have, however, been numerous reports where lymphocytes from the normal donors or from close relatives of melanoma patients have shown high degrees of cytotoxicity against melanoma cell lines and in some reports antibody has also been shown to be present in such so-called controls (Hellström, Hellström, Sjögren *et al.*, 1973; Morton,

1971). Studies are in progress in the authors' laboratory to grade the degree of immunological reactivity of non-melanoma individuals with varying exposure to either patients with melanoma or melanoma tissue, in the hope that this will clarify the so-called false positive results.

Another aspect of the specificity of the tumour antigens relates to the types of tumour antigen demonstrated. It is now clear that we are not dealing with single antigenic changes or alterations in tumour cells and that these cells can contain varying types of antigen, against which different components of the immune response may be demonstrated. There appears to be antigen(s) on the surface of melanoma cells which are individually specific and demonstrable both by immunofluorescence and by complement-dependent cytotoxicity. The evidence for individual specificity in melanoma is summarised in Table 10.6 (Lewis *et al.*, 1976). In addition, there must be some degree of group specific or common antigen on the surface of the cell which can be

Table 10.6   Evidence for individually specific antigen in Melanoma

Lewis Lewis *et al.*	1967b 1969	No cross-reactivity with complement-dependent serum cytotoxicity
Lewis *et al.*	1969	Stronger autologous than allogeneic reactions by membrane immuno-fluorescence
Lewis *et al.*	1971	Presence of anti-idiotypic anti-antibody
Lewis and Phillips	1972a	Failure of allogeneic cells to absorb completely antibody
Lewis and Phillips	1972b	Ability to separate effects of autologous antibody from allogeneic anti-cytoplasmic antibody
Lewis *et al.*	1975	Differences in antibody response to auto- and allo-immunization
Bodurtha	1975	No cross-reactivity with complement-dependent serum cytotoxicity

demonstrated by lymphocytotoxicity most clearly in melanoma cell lines and by very weak reactions using the patient's serum or allogeneic serum. Fetal antigens (Alexander, 1972) have also been detected in a number of tumour systems (Gold and Freedman, 1965; Coggin and Anderson, 1974) and also in malignant melanoma (Avis and Lewis, 1973), but these have been shown to be distinctly different from the other surface antigens and may or may not be immunogenic to the host bearing the tumour. The cytoplastic contents of melanoma cells also exhibit antigens which are different from the surface membrane components so far described. There is an element of group specificity when these antigens are examined by serological means and antibody directed against these internal antigens has a different time relationship with the stage of disease to that described for antibody against the membrane antigens (Lewis, Avis, Phillips *et al.*, 1973). This particular antibody response will be discussed in more detail in a later section.

The possibility that some of the cytoplasmic antigens may be related to viral antigens has recently been brought to light by the work of Birkmayer and his colleagues, who have demonstrated the presence of reverse transcriptase in melanoma cell preparations (Birkmayer, Balda and Miller, 1974; Birkmayer *et al.*, 1975; Parsons, Goss and Pope, 1974). This is at present an area of considerably interesting research.

McBride and his colleagues have also demonstrated antibodies directed against nuclear and nucleolar components of melanoma cells and have shown a different relationship between the antibodies directed against these antigens and the stage of the disease (McBride, Bowen and Dmochowski, 1972). The various melanoma antigens so far described are summarised in Figure 10.16.

The cytoplasmic antigens certainly appear to be the ones that cause the most confusion and controversy in the literature and it is of some importance that investigators working on melanoma antigens or any tumour antigens should specify which antigen is being studied and be aware of these differences to avoid confusion in comparisons.

THE RELATIONSHIP BETWEEN THE RESPONSE TO MELANOMA ANTIGEN AND THE NATURAL HISTORY OF MELANOMA

The only certain way of knowing whether any *in vitro* procedure has any real value is to show that it can explain some facet of the natural history of the disease under consideration. It is a continued study of the natural history of the disease which will prevent above all

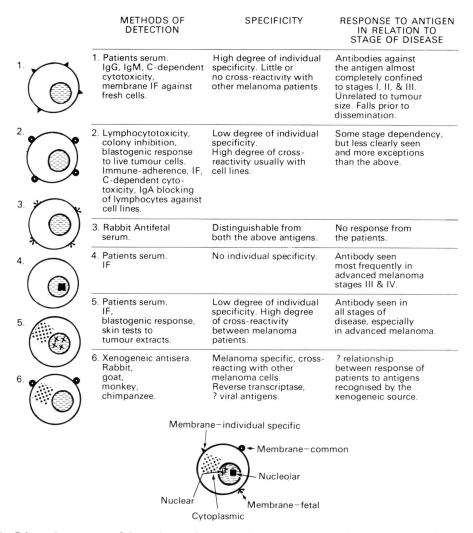

	METHODS OF DETECTION	SPECIFICITY	RESPONSE TO ANTIGEN IN RELATION TO STAGE OF DISEASE
1.	1. Patients serum. IgG, IgM, C-dependent cytotoxicity, membrane IF against fresh cells.	High degree of individual specificity. Little or no cross-reactivity with other melanoma patients.	Antibodies against the antigen almost completely confined to stages I, II, & III. Unrelated to tumour size. Falls prior to dissemination.
2.	2. Lymphocytotoxicity, colony inhibition, blastogenic response to live tumour cells. Immune-adherence, IF, C-dependent cyto-toxicity, IgA blocking of lymphocytes against cell lines.	Low degree of individual specificity. High degree of cross-reactivity usually with cell lines.	Some stage dependency, but less clearly seen and more exceptions than the above.
3.	3. Rabbit Antifetal serum.	Distinguishable from both the above antigens.	No response from the patients.
4.	4. Patients serum. IF	No individual specificity.	Antibody seen most frequently in advanced melanoma stages III & IV.
5.	5. Patients serum. IF, blastogenic response, skin tests to tumour extracts.	Low degree of individual specificity. High degree of cross-reactivity between melanoma patients.	Antibody seen in all stages of disease, especially in advanced melanoma.
6.	6. Xenogeneic antisera. Rabbit, goat, monkey, chimpanzee.	Melanoma specific, cross-reacting with other melanoma cells. Reverse transcriptase, ? viral antigens.	? relationship between response of patients to antigens recognised by the xenogeneic source.

Membrane—individual specific

Membrane—common

Nucleolar

Membrane—fetal

Nuclear

Cytoplasmic

Fig. 10.16   Schematic summary of the various melanoma antigens described and the methods of their detection.

else the following of artefacts and the production of theories that have no substance. As quoted by Sir David Smithers in a symposium of the British Cancer Council in 1971 '... we would do well to pay attention to those Scottish physicians in 1802 and abandon theories which a correct history of the disease denies' (Smithers, 1971). Here again malignant melanoma is a unique tumour to study from an immunological point of view, since the natural history is well understood as will be seen from the extensive coverage in the remainder of this book.

The question, therefore, must be answered: do any of these tests for tumour antigen, antibody or cell-mediated immunity have any relationship to the staging of the disease and do they have any prognostic value? It is perhaps reasonable to start with evidence of humoral immunity since it was the observation that antibody in the serum of patients in Uganda with Burkitt's lymphoma and melanoma appeared to be controlling their tumours and not in those that have rapid spread, that first led to this particular approach (Klein *et al.*, 1966; Lewis, 1967b). There is now ample evidence from a number of series that the presence of some tumour antibodies in melanoma, particularly those directed against the membrane of the living cells, can be shown to be stage-related. They are found predominantly in either stage I or II, rarely in III and practically never in stage IV. This relationship is most clearly seen for those antibodies which are directed against the surface membrane of the autologous cells. These antibodies have been shown to be complement-dependent (Lewis, 1967b; Bodurtha *et al.*, 1975; Canevari *et al.*, 1975). It is, however, also clear that there are circulating antibodies which do not have such a clear-cut relationship with the stage of the disease and it is the failure to distinguish these other types of antibody response which has been responsible for some of the confusion and apparent controversies. There is increasing evidence that antibodies may be produced against the internal components of tumour cells and that the liberation of such disrupted cell contents may produce antibody responses which persist as long as the stimulus is present. It is probable that this response is not of a protective nature in the individual, since these antibodies would not react against the surface of circulating autologous cells and, therefore, would have no clear relationship to the early stage of the disease versus the late stage (Lewis, Hartmann and Jerry, 1976). This will be discussed in more detail in a later section on mechanisms of failure.

Several studies have indicated that as the disease progresses a fall in antimembrane or complement-dependent cytotoxic antibodies precedes the appearance of widespread metastases (Lewis *et al.*, 1969; Bodurtha *et al.*, 1975). The presence of these antibodies cannot be related to the volume or size of the tumour in the patient and is, therefore, not related to tumour load but to the degree of localisation or dissemination of the tumour (Lewis,

McCloy and Blake, 1973). This was emphasised by comparisons between individuals who had large amounts of local tumour and had positive antibody and those with disseminated but very small volumes of tumour which were clearly antibody-negative. These earlier results have recently been confirmed by other groups (Bodurtha *et al.*, 1975; Canevari *et al.*, 1975). The relationship between antimembrane and anticytoplasmic antibodies and the course of the disease is summarised in Figure 10.17. The possible significance and implications of these findings will be discussed later.

The situation regarding cell-mediated immunity and the natural history of the disease is perhaps less clear, but again there is a strong tendency for the reactions to be most clearly demonstrated in the early stages and less demonstrable as the disease progresses. Although there are variations and some authors using methods of measurement of some forms of cell-mediated immunity have shown that this is not the case (De Vries, Rümke and Bernheim, 1972; Hellström, Hellström, Sjögren *et al.*, 1971; Nairn, 1974; Veronesi *et al.*, 1973), others have demonstrated that there is a stage relationship (Butterworth *et al.*, 1974; Currie, Lejeune and Hamilton-Fairley, 1971; Hellström, Warner, Hellström *et al.*, 1973; Mackie *et al.*, 1972). Perhaps one of the most recent examples is the combined study previously mentioned between a group in the U.S.A. and the U.S.S.R. where use was made of a purified glycolipoprotein from the surface of melanoma cells. They demonstrated that the reactivity in individual patients was most frequently seen in early stage disease and less frequently seen in late stage disease (Gorodilova and Hollinshead, 1975). These distinctions are by no means absolute and reflect the relative lack of precision in most of the tests of cell-mediated immunity, as compared to those for humoral immunity. There are other explanations in which some aspects of cellular response to these tumour antigens may persist independently of other reactions of the host.

Although the major emphasis has been to demonstrate the effect on peripheral blood

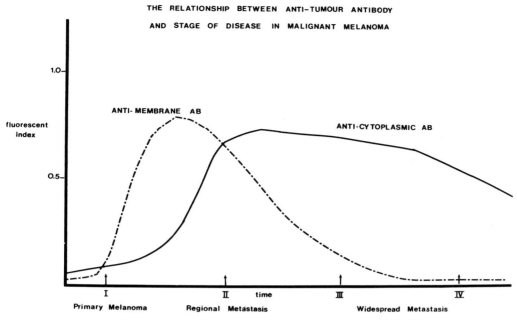

Fig. 10.17   Time relationship between two antimelanoma antibody systems and the natural history of the disease.

components of the immune system, attempts have been made to analyse the effects of lymphocytes from draining lymph nodes in tumours, both in experimental animals (Alexander, Bensted and Delorme, 1967) and more recently in human melanoma (Nind *et al.*, 1973). Nairn (1974) reported that the cells from draining lymph nodes were less cytotoxic than the peripheral blood lymphocytes, but of course here one is dealing with different populations of cells. There is some evidence from our own studies that cells from draining lymph nodes in over 30 patients with melanoma had no relationship at all to the levels of cytotoxic lymphocytes in the peripheral blood. The critical study is to compare the draining lymph nodes with non-draining lymph nodes.

In summary, therefore, one can make the general statement that immune reactivity of the patient against his own tumour is most clearly seen in the early stage of malignancy and either less clearly seen or not seen at all

as the disease progresses (Fig. 10.18). This change in reactivity varies with individual patients and individual tumours, and in making this statement the exceptions must be borne in mind. In melanoma the evidence would suggest that measures of cell-mediated immunity, with the exception of some of the tests like the LAI, appear to become unreactive somewhere between stage II and III. This would imply not inherent failure or non-responsiveness of the immune system, but an acquired failure of immune response during the evolution of the malignant process. If this is the case then mechanisms must exist to explain this acquired failure and these will now be considered in some detail. It is worth emphasising also that the relationship between the immune system and the progression of an established tumour may well be considerably different from the mechanism that may or may not operate in the induction period of such neoplasms.

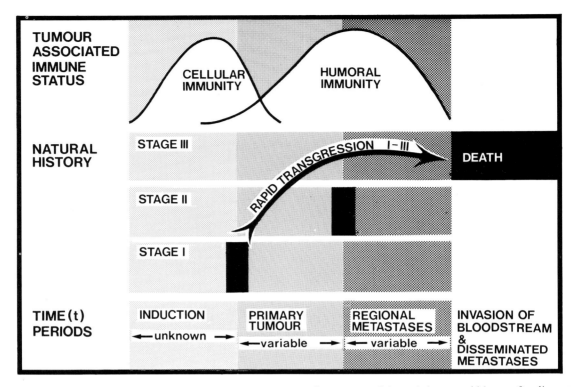

Fig. 10.18   Schematic summary of relationship between tumour immune reactivity and the natural history of malignant melanoma. (*From* Lewis, 1973b)

REASONS AND MECHANISMS FOR FAILURE OF IMMUNE CONTROL OF TUMOURS

Although this has become a very exciting and central area of tumour immunology, it is important to have a clear picture of which aspect of the malignant process and which element of the immune response one is considering in order to avoid confusion. A growing primary tumour, the regional lymph node metastases, the blood borne spread of metastatic cells and the continued growth and tertiary development of established metastases, all present different challenges to an immune system, whose reactivity differs during these various advances of malignancy. The growing awareness that some form of blockade of the immune response occurs in malignancy has been one which has generated considerable in-

vestigative effort (Mastrangelo, Laucius and Outzen, 1975). The central problem, however, is the nature of such blocking factors. Many have been described and possibly more than one or all of them exist, but they are present at different stages of the malignant development. The various mechanisms so far described are summarised for simplicity in the following diagram (Fig. 10.19).

Here again, emphasis must be placed on the type of tumour and host examined in such a situation. It becomes clear that if one is dealing with a lymphoma or leukaemia where the central immune system itself is involved in the malignant process, this will make the situation somewhat different from a solid tumour presenting a challenge to an otherwise intact immunity.

In this respect malignant melanoma is, again, a very important tumour in that the vari-

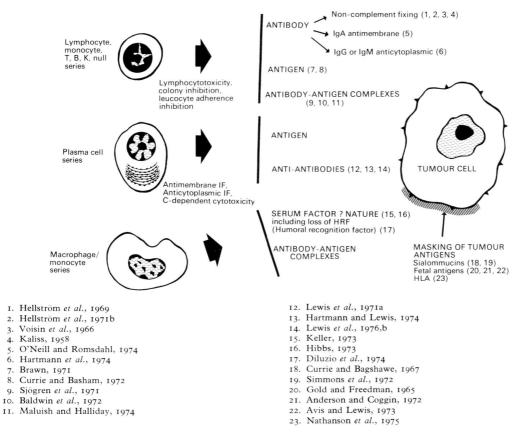

Fig. 10.19   Concepts of blocking of antitumour immune reactions in malignancy.

1. Hellström et al., 1969
2. Hellström et al., 1971b
3. Voisin et al., 1966
4. Kaliss, 1958
5. O'Neill and Romsdahl, 1974
6. Hartmann et al., 1974
7. Brawn, 1971
8. Currie and Basham, 1972
9. Sjögren et al., 1971
10. Baldwin et al., 1972
11. Maluish and Halliday, 1974

12. Lewis et al., 1971a
13. Hartmann and Lewis, 1974
14. Lewis et al., 1976,b
15. Keller, 1973
16. Hibbs, 1973
17. Diluzio et al., 1974
18. Currie and Bagshawe, 1967
19. Simmons et al., 1972
20. Gold and Freedman, 1965
21. Anderson and Coggin, 1972
22. Avis and Lewis, 1973
23. Nathanson et al., 1975

ous stages of immune stimulation and abnormality can be studied and dissected out in detail.

Various examples of immune blocking in malignancy have been extensively reviewed in recent publications (Mastrangelo, Laucius and Outzen 1975). One of the possible mechanisms is some form of masking of tumour antigens, thus allowing the tumour to bypass the immune system. To some extent this has been shown in neoplasms such as choricarcinoma (Currie and Bagshawe, 1967) and in some well-defined animal tumours, but even in the animal models this is not a universal mechanism and the evidence for such masking of surface antigens is not completely established in all human tumours. This idea has been used in some

forms of immunotherapy by treating the tumour cells with neuraminidase in an attempt to clear various forms of sialomucins from the tumour cell surfaces (Simmons and Rios, 1971; Seigler et al., 1972; Seigler et al., 1973).

The role of carcinoembryonic or fetal antigens certainly has been examined in this light (Coggin and Anderson, 1974; Baldwin, Glaves and Vose, 1974b) and the concept that fetal antigens might mask tumour antigens and render the tumour less immunogenic to the host is certainly one worthy of consideration. Once again, this has not been shown to be the universal situation and in fact in melanoma, fetal antigens have been shown to be distinctly different from the tumour specific antigens. The two antigens can exist and can be demonstrated at the same time using serological means, so that at least the humoral immune system still recognises the tumour antigens at the same time (Avis and Lewis, 1973; Rowden and Lewis, 1975b). The fact that both colony-inhibiting lymphocytes and cytotoxic lymphocytes have also been demonstrated against fresh as well as cultured tumour cells makes this mechanism even less likely, but has not been entirely ruled out.

The next consideration is the role of so-called blocking antibody, and at one stage this was considered to be a likely mechanism for prevention of effective contact between cytotoxic lymphocytes and tumour cells. Antibody could combine on the surface of cells without fixing complement, thus not killing the cell and yet preventing the lymphocytes from doing so (Hellström et al., 1969). O'Neill and Romsdahl (1974), in a recent report, demonstrated in 9 of 10 patients with melanoma the presence of an IgA antibody which blocked lymphocytotoxicity against a melanoma cell line. The phenomenon of blocking of various aspects of cell-mediated immunity by serum factors has been extensively reported by a number of observers, using colony-inhibition (Hellström, Sjögren, Warner, et al., 1971; Heppner et al., 1973), cytotoxicity of lymphocytes (Sjögren et al., 1971; Voisin, Kinsky and Jansen, 1966) and the leucocyte adherence test (Maluish and Halliday, 1974; Hartmann et al., 1974). The nature of the blocking factors is still under considerable debate. Some investigators emphasise the role of antitumour antibody, others immune complexes, and others tumour antigen. The main concepts are summarised in Figure 10.19. Theoretically there is no reason why any one of these should not be applicable. In fact, the possibility exists that all of these mechanisms may operate in different forms at different stages of the disease, and that the arguments really result from different groups studying different tumour/host relationships. In some studies, tumour nodules were treated by an elution procedure which isolated immunoglobulin thought to be specific for the tumours in question (Sjögren et al., 1972). These results have two implications, one being that this demonstrates at least an aspect of blocking in the local tumour nodule and the second, the ability of growing tumours to soak up antibody from the circulation. This argument has been further supported by claims of immunoglobulin bound on tumour cells in vivo (Witz, 1973); Romsdahl and Cox, 1971). Other reports, however, have related the eluted immunoglobulin to the presence of host cells infiltrating the tumour, particularly lymphocytes and plasma cells, and in some cases monocytes and macrophages (Roberts et al., 1973; Johansson and Ljungovist, 1974). This illustrates one of the dangers of assuming that a tumour is a homogeneous mass of tumour cells, when in certain circumstances, particularly lymph node involvement or tumours in body cavities, the component of host cells may well form a major part of the mass of the tumour at any one time. The ability, for instance, of macrophages to occupy a considerable part of tumour nodules has been emphasised by a number of investigators and beautifully demonstrated by Lejeune and his colleagues in the mouse melanoma system (Lejeune, 1973).

Another line of investigation was directed towards elucidating the reason for alterations in the levels of circulating antibodies during tumour progression. Since the antimembrane antibodies and the cytotoxic antibodies were not related to the volume or mass of tumour and appeared to fall prior to dissemination (Lewis, McCloy and Blake, 1973), the likelihood of the tumour soaking up such an antibody was considered unlikely, and indeed this has been confirmed (Bodurtha et al., 1975). Several studies have indicated that antibody does not simply soak into the tumour and become attached to the tumour cells. In some recent investigations, it was demonstrated that serum antibody levels had no relationship to the antibody on tumour cell surfaces in solid tumours and most of the immunoglobulin in solid tumour was seen on plasma cells and B cells (Lewis, Proctor, Thomson, et al., 1976), or monocytes or macrophages (Proctor et al., 1976). During these investigations it was shown that a negative serum in some melanoma patients could specifically block the autologous positive serum at a different moment of time in the same individual. This appeared to be an IgG antibody in which no antigen component could be detected. The suggestion was made that this was an anti-idiotypic antibody directed against the individually specific antitumour antibody. It is of some interest that anti-idiotypic antibodies have subsequently been suggested as an important component in the role of immune regulation and control (Jerne, 1974).

As a result of these initial studies, other forms of anti-antibody have been demonstrated, particularly in human malignant melanoma. These are summarised in Figure 10.20 and include anti-antibodies directed against the variable region (the so-called anti-idiotypic antibodies) (Lewis, Phillips, Cook *et al.*, 1971), those directed against the hinge region (the anti-(Fab¹)$_2$ antibodies), and finally those directed against the Fc portion (the anti-

Fc or rheumatoid-like factors). The anti-(Fab¹)$_2$ antibodies have been shown to be directed against the anticytoplasmic antimelanoma antibody and are believed to be an attempt of the immune system to clear these inappropriate and ineffective antibodies from the system. The demonstration by Cano and others in the authors' laboratory of immune complexes in the sera of the same patients indicate that they may be one of the mechanisms for producing both the anti-Fab and the anti-Fc antibodies described (Jerry *et al.*, 1976; Cano *et al.*, 1976). Viza and his colleagues (1975) have also recently demonstrated the presence of melanoma antigen in the serum of some of these patients, which does not correlate with the disappearance of antimembrane antibodies or cytotoxic lymphocytes, but is most clearly seen in patients with very advanced disease where no aspect of immunity can be easily measured. This latter observation

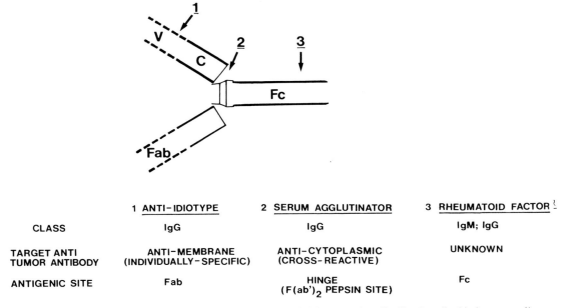

ANTI-ANTIBODY SYSTEMS IN MELANOMA

	1 ANTI-IDIOTYPE	2 SERUM AGGLUTINATOR	3 RHEUMATOID FACTOR
CLASS	IgG	IgG	IgM; IgG
TARGET ANTI TUMOR ANTIBODY	ANTI-MEMBRANE (INDIVIDUALLY-SPECIFIC)	ANTI-CYTOPLASMIC (CROSS-REACTIVE)	UNKNOWN
ANTIGENIC SITE	Fab	HINGE (F(ab')$_2$ PEPSIN SITE)	Fc

Fig. 10.20   Diagram of immunoglobulin G and sites of action of different anti-antibodies described in human malignancy.

is hardly surprising since patients with very advanced malignant melanoma may well have deeply pigmented skin and even melanuria.

The presence of immune complexes and particularly anti-immunoglobulins have been shown in a number of chronic disease states where persistent antigenic stimulation occurs, such as in chronic Gram-positive infections, in parasitic disorders such as malaria and leprosy and in rheumatoid arthritis and related auto-immune phenomena. These, in common with malignancy, illustrate the derangement of immune regulation and control following a persistent stimulation of an antigen, without its removal from the system. This is a way of looking at lack of immune control in malignancy from a slightly different point of view (Lewis, Hartmann and Jerry, 1976). Another aspect of

immune derangement can be seen in renal glomerular deposition of immune complexes resulting in the nephrotic syndrome (Loughridge and Lewis, 1971). This complication of malignancy has been reported by a number of investigators and the subject recently reviewed (Lancet, 1975). The complexes have been eluted from kidneys under such circumstances and shown to contain antitumour antibodies (Lewis, Loughridge and Phillips, 1971), a situation confirmed in experimental animals (Poskitt, Poskitt and Wallace, 1974; Mac-Fadden, Lewis and Rowden, 1976). Minor degrees of renal deposition of antibody–antigen may well be more frequent than the recorded incidence of nephrosis indicates. In several recent autopsies in patients with melanoma, immune complexes have been

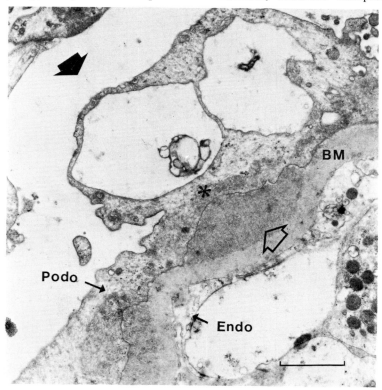

Fig. 10.21   Electron micrograph of part of a capillary loop in a glomerulus. Electron dense material (*open arrow*) is present in the basement membrane (BM). Associated densities (⋆) are seen in the overlying fused podocyte foot processes (Podo). Close arrow indicates urinary space; Endothelium (Endo), ×28 300 (1 micron marker)
Material—Autopsy kidney from terminal malignant melanoma patient.

identified including the third component of complement (Fig. 10.21). This phenomenon should be kept in mind when various forms of immunotherapy are considered, particularly passive transfer of allogeneic or xenogeneic antisera.

Studies on the effects of growing tumours on the regional lymph nodes clearly may be of considerable importance in this understanding of immune derangement. It has been known for some time that the draining lymph nodes in an area of growing tumour may be abnormal (Alexander *et al.*, 1967) and several authors have shown some expression of this in terms of *in vitro* testing of lymph node cells (Nind *et al.*, 1973). In addition, there have been some reports showing the increased presence of immunoglobulin-positive cells in such lymph nodes (Ritchers and Kaspersky, 1975; Lewis, Proctor, Thomson *et al.*, 1976), and the nature of this immune blockade in such tissue may well throw further light on the progression of these tumours and their ability to become widely metastatic.

IMMUNOLOGICAL MANIPULATIONS (IMMUNOTHERAPY)

The ultimate objective of the study of tumour immunology is to produce some form of therapeutic effect. This is, again, by no means a new subject and as Currie (1972) has pointed out in a review of 80 years of immunotherapy, was strongly suggested around the turn of the century. Lack of success at this time resulted in an almost complete abandonment for a number of years. Hamilton-Fairley in a lecture to the Royal College of Physicians in London in 1969 pointed out that three eras occurred—the initial era of optimism, where everyone with a syringe and some mice tried immunotherapy, followed by an era of pessimism, where all seemed to have failed, and finally, the era of realism, hopefully the present time. There has, however, recently been a tremendous upsurge in enthusiasm and interest in this concept (Mastrangelo, Berd and Bellet, 1976). Once again malignant melanoma has played a fairly major role amongst tumours

studied in this respect, and there are several recent extensive reviews of this subject. The main references to immunotherapy of human malignant melanoma are summarised in Tables 7 to 12.

The methods of such immune stimulation can be conveniently divided into two major categories: (1) non-specific immune stimulation, i.e. the use of methods of stimulating immunity with the hope that in addition tumour-directed immune reactions will result, and (2) a specific immune stimulation in an attempt to produce a response which will be largely, if not completely, tumour directed. Once again, to have a rational basis for this important therapy, one must have a clear picture of which aspect of malignancy it is hoped to combat and, therefore, which type of immune response should be produced. More often than not, the attempts at immunotherapy have not taken these facts into consideration and have been, therefore, largely either anecdotal or in many cases performed in a rather blind fashion.

Non-specific immunotherapy

Non-specific immunotherapy can be divided into local tumour manipulations and general immune stimulation.

LOCAL IMMUNOTHERAPY

Local immunotherapy goes back to the era of Coley and his colleagues who attempted the direct inoculation of products of certain bacteria into human tumours. More recently it has been extended by the use of agents such as vaccinia virus and the intralesional injection of BCG organisms. This latter approach has been used extensively, with most series showing local effect in that the tumours were replaced with lymphocytes and monocytes (Lieberman, Wybran and Epstein, 1975) and in many cases disappeared, but few reports indicate regression of non-injected lesions, though this has occasionally been claimed. Unfortunately, serious complications can result from this approach and there have now been well-documented series where severe systemic effects of the BCG bacillus have been noted (Serrow *et al.*, 1975) with some deaths (Sparks *et al.*, 1973).

Another approach pioneered by Edmund

Klein (1969) and his colleagues has been to sensitise patients with DNCB and, after the development of a hypersensitivity reaction, to treat the local skin tumour with another dose of the same agent, resulting in an enhanced hypersensitivity reaction which included the destruction of the tumour nodules.

Some years ago Finney, Byers and Wilson (1969) showed that antitumour antibodies raised by immunising patients with tumour homogenates and adjuvant could then, by injection into tumour nodules cause temporary regression. All these forms of local attack on the tumour have one major drawback and that

is that they do not interact with the metastatic cells which in many instances are the main problem. They do, however, have a place in local management of patients with skin metastases, particularly in melanoma. Table 10.7 summarises the main references in the use of local immunotherapy of melanoma.

GENERAL NON-SPECIFIC IMMUNOTHERAPY

This approach includes the use of immune stimulants such as BCG and *Corynebacterium parvum* and more recently interest has centred around a drug called levamisole, which appears to be not so much an immunostimulant as an

Table 10.7 Approaches to immunisation in malignant melanoma

Non-specific—local

Coley	1893	Bacterial products	Destruction of local tumour with inflammation
Pack	1950	Rabies vaccination	Increased survival for more than 10 years in an individual
Burdick	1960		
Burdick and Hawk	1964		Variable degree of local response and effect on non-injected nodules
Milton and Lane Brown	1966		
Hunter-Craig et al.	1970	Vaccinia injection	Only lesion injected disappeared
McCarthy and Milton	1975		Disappearance of metastatic skin nodules in addition to those injected
Everall et al.	1975		Increased survival after injecting primary melanoma prior to surgical excision
Roenigk et al.	1975		
Stjernsward and Levin	1971		
Klein and Holterman	1972	DCNB	
Malek-Mansour et al.	1973		
Tisman et al.	1975		
Klein et al.	1975	DCNB and PPD	
Morton et al.	1971		
Krementz et al.	1971		
Nathanson	1972	BCG intralesional	
Seigler et al.	1972		
Klein et al.	1973	BCG and PPD	
Sparks et al.	1973	BCG	
Pinsky et al.	1973		
Smith et al.	1973	BCG intratumoral injection	
Baker and Taub	1973a		
Minton	1973	BCG and mumps virus in metastatic melanoma	
Grant et al.	1974	BCG	
Lieberman et al.	1974	BCG with histological and immunological changes	
Levy et al.	1974	BCG	
Mastrangelo et al.	1975b	BCG regression of pulmonary metastases	
Mastrangelo et al.	1975c	BCG	
Lieberman et al.	1975	BCG with histological and immunological changes	
Seigler, Shingleton and Pickrell	1975	Intralesional BCG plus immune lymphocytes intravenously and neuraminidase-treated melanoma cells	

immunoregulator and, therefore, has some interesting potential (Amery, 1976).

The most widely reported non-specific immune stimulant in malignancy and melanoma in particular is BCG (*Bacillus Calmette-Guérin*), a modified bovine tubercle bacillus described originally by Calmette and Guérin. Several investigations pointed to its potential use in adjuvant immunotherapy. In the first instance this was suggested by the observations of Halpern *et al.* (1959) and Old, Clarke and Benacerraf (1959) that the progression of experimental tumours in rats and mice could be influenced by administration of BCG and, secondly, the clinical effects noted by Mathè and his group in human leukaemia (Mathè *et al.*, 1968). Further support comes from the observations made by Davignon and his colleagues that the incidence of leukaemia in children receiving BCG was decreased (Davignon *et al.*, 1970). The use of BCG in human melanoma has been extensively reviewed during the past few years (Baker and Taub, 1973b; Nathanson, 1974; Mastrangelo, Laucius and Outzen, 1975; Gutterman *et al.*, 1975a). The

material has been used as intradermal injections, scarification of the skin, orally, and by the intraperitoneal route.

Several groups using BCG in melanoma patients have claimed increase in disease-free intervals and the signs of alteration in the progression of melanoma (Blumming, Vogel and Ziegler, 1972; Gutterman *et al.*, 1973a; Ikonopisov, 1975; Currie and McElwain, 1975). The main reports in the literature related to the use of immune adjuvants in melanoma are summarised in Table 10.8.

Specific immunotherapy

Specific immunotherapy can be considered under three headings: passive, adoptive and active.

PASSIVE SPECIFIC IMMUNOTHERAPY

This largely consists of transfusion of blood or plasma from individuals who were apparently recovering or recovered from their tumours, into those whose tumours were progressing (Horn and Horn, 1971). Although

Table 10.8 Immunotherapy of malignant melanoma

Non-specific—general (BCG; scarification or intradermal injection; *C. parvum*; Levamisole; PHA, etc.)

Lewis, Humble *et al.*	1971	IV PHA (phytohaemagglutinin). Partial regression of melanoma with coating of tumour with antibody
Israel and Halpern	1972	*C. parvum*
Blumming, Vogel and Ziegler	1972	BCG—comparison of 2 modes of administration
Currie	1973	BCG
Klein *et al.*	1973	BCG
Gutterman *et al.*	1973a	BCG in metastatic disease
Gutterman *et al.*	1973b	BCG and immune reactions
Israel and Edelstein	1973	*C. parvum*
Morton *et al.*	1974	BCG—summary of 7 years' experience
Ikonopisov	1975	BCG—increase in disease-free intervals
Lewis *et al.*	1975	Oral BCG with or without auto-immunisation
Gutterman *et al.*	1975b	BCG in recurrent melanoma
Lewis *et al.*	1975	Levamisole—compared with BCG
McCulloch *et al.*	1975	BCG—improved survival
Shibata *et al.*	1976	Oral BCG with or without auto- or allo-immunisation
Shibata *et al.*	1976	Levamisole—effect on antibodies production
Lewis, Proctor *et al.*	1976	IV PHA—partial regression of melanoma with coating of tumour with antibody

there have been occasional claims of success, most investigators would regard this as being of limited value and may even be of danger, in view of the possibility of enhancement and also the potential risk of an immune complex disease. It is well established that antibody–antigen complexes may be deposited not only in the reticuloendothelial system in individuals with malignancy, but also on the basement membrane of the kidneys with the possible relationship to the nephrotic syndrome (Loughridge and Lewis, 1971; Lewis, Loughridge and Phillips, 1971).

More recently Ghose and his colleagues following up an older concept have attempted to use antisera raised in other species such as goats and then couple the goat antimelanoma antibodies to chlorambucil, in an attempt to use the specificity of the antibody and the cytotoxic effect of chemotherapeutic agent. Some controversy, however, exists concerning whether chlorambucil really does remain firmly attached to the antibody or whether this is merely a synergistic effect rather than a carrying effect of antibody (Vennegoor and Van Smeerdijk, 1975; Gutterman *et al.*, 1975a). The use of heteroantisera alone has also been attempted using serum raised in rabbits, chimpanzees, and numerous xenogeneic hosts (Mann, 1975).

ADOPTIVE IMMUNOTHERAPY

In addition, either allogeneic or xenogeneic lymphocytes have also been transfused into individuals with malignancy with variable responses. The tremendous danger of graft versus host reactivity in these patients is one of the major drawbacks and limits this approach considerably. All of these methods have in common one major disadvantage and that is that the procedure does not take into account the patient's own responsiveness or lack of responsiveness to the tumour and does nothing to alter the immune status of the host. The next approach of adoptive specific immunotherapy does take these problems into consideration and various procedures have been used including cross-immunisation and cross-transfusion of either lymphocytes or serum, i.e. immunising two patients with each other's tumours and then cross-transfusing. This is in a sense a combination of passive and adoptive immunotherapy (Mansell, Krementz and Diluzio, 1975) and although it may sound promising it has certainly not produced the successes that would indicate it to be of major importance.

Other procedures have included taking the patient's lymphocytes and altering their reactivity by exposure to tumours or tumour antigens followed by reinfusing them into the individual (Nadler and Moore, 1965; Oon, Butterworth *et al.*, 1975). In addition, lymphocytes have been exposed *in vitro* to phytohaemagglutinin (PHA), and then reinjected into another patient. In more recent times, two potentially more exciting approaches to adoptive immunotherapy have been used, one following on the discovery of transfer factor by Lawrence (1963). This substance of low molecular weight and obtained from lymphocytes can be injected into another host and transfer immunological reactivity. This approach has been used in immunotherapy of malignant melanoma by a number of groups (Oettgen, Old and Boyse, 1971; Spitler *et al.*, 1972; Brandes, Galton and Wiltshaw, 1971), again with limited success. The procedure is to immunise either another individual or another animal, obtain lymphocytes, extract transfer factor, then inject this into the patient with malignancy. In other approaches, use is made of so-called immune RNA which is similar in principle to transfer factor, but is the actual RNA from stimulated lymphocytes. This may be administered to patients and can apparently then stimulate the host's lymphoid system to respond to the antigens which stimulated the original donor lymphocytes, from which the RNA was obtained (Fishman, 1961; Decker and Pilch, 1972).

This has been extensively explored by Pilch and his colleagues and they have reported some changes in patients with malignant melanoma (Pilch, Fritze and Kerne, 1975). The various series using passive and adoptive immunotherapy in melanoma are shown in Tables 10.9 and 10.10.

Table 10.9   Immunotherapy of malignant melanoma

Specific—passive

Sumner and Foraker	1960	Allogeneic sera transfused into melanoma patient
Teimourian and McCune	1963	
Stephens	1966	
Ghose et al.	1972	Xenogeneic antisera and chlorambucil
Ghose et al.	1975	
Oon, Apsey et al.	1975	Autologous immunisation and then coupled with chlorambucil and reinfused. Some control of advanced melanoma and altered immune reactions

Table 10.10   Adoptive immunotherapy

Nadler and Moore	1969	Leucocyte transfusion with or without cross immunisation with allogeneic cells
Frenster and Rogoway	1970	In vitro activation of lymphocytes with tumour antigen and reinfusion
Moore and Gerner	1971	Large-scale tissue culture of lymphocytes and reinfusion
Krementz et al.	1971	Leucocyte transusion with or without cross immunisation with allogeneic cells
Curtis	1971	
Brandes et al.	1971	Transfer factor
Spitler et al.	1973	
Golub and Morton	1974	In vitro activation of lymphocytes with tumour antigen and reinfusion
Pilch et al.	1974	Xenogeneic immune RNA
Seigler, Shingleton and Pickrell	1975	
Seigler, Shingleton, Horn et al.	1975	Autologous lymphocytes co-cultured with auto- or allogeneic tumour cells then reinjected into patient
Oon, Butterworth et al.	1975	Allo-immunisation and transfusion of lymphocytes to melanoma patients. Clinical improvement plus changes in antitumour immunity

ACTIVE SPECIFIC IMMUNOTHERAPY

This is possibly the oldest approach to immunotherapy and yet the one which has in some respects the greatest appeal. It goes directly to the problem of using the patient's tumour to stimulate the individual, in the hope of a response against the tumour.

Use of tumour vaccines as previously stated is a method that was in vogue many years ago and went into disrepute. It has, however, been recently re-examined by a number of groups. Several reports have shown that immune responsiveness can be temporarily restored in patients who are immunised with their own tumour cells (Humphrey, Lincoln and Griffen, 1968; Ikonopisov et al., 1970; Currie et al., 1971). In addition, combinations of auto-immunisation with and without BCG or other non-specific stimulants have also been investigated. In addition, allo-immunisation of mel-

anoma patients is being looked at by a number of groups. In many situations the time when immunotherapy is likely to be more successful, that is when there is minimal disease, is the time when it is least possible to obtain sufficient tumour for auto-immunisation procedures. Therefore, combinations of non-specific immune stimulation and specific would seem reasonable, and there have been a number of reports that BCG given with tumour inocula reduced the number of tumour cells needed to produce a particular level of cytotoxic lymphocytes or antibody (Currie, 1973). Auto-immunisation given into a lymph node area where BCG scarification was performed appears also to increase reactivity (Gutterman et al., 1973b).

There have been several reports showing that BCG alone is not very successful in producing either cytotoxic lymphocytes or antibody, but there have been other studies showing that BCG can cause a re-emergence of both antibody and lymphocytes following auto-immunisation (Lewis, Jerry and Shibata, 1975; Shibata et al., 1976) (Fig. 10.22). There have also been suggestions that levamisole may function in this respect in restoring normal immune reactivity so that immunisation will be more effective (Amery, 1976).

Combined chemotherapy and immunotherapy

Finally, the approach of using chemotherapy and immunotherapy in combination has been perhaps one of the most exciting recent developments. Several groups have shown that combinations of chemotherapeutic agents, particularly DTIC (imidazole carboxa-

mide), used in patients who are also being treated either with BCG, levamisole or immunisation procedures, result in arrest of tumour progression, even in established malignancy (Gutterman et al., 1975b; Israel and Halpern, 1972; Ikonopisov, 1975; Gutterman et al., 1974; McCarthy and Milton, 1975). It is perhaps too early to state categorically that this is the best approach to the problem but certainly at the moment it is the most promising (Table 10.12). Whether this combined approach works because of a synergistic effect between the cytopathic effect of chemotherapy and the immune system both working together on the tumour, or whether the chemotherapy may in fact alter the derangement of the immune system and allow immunotherapy to be effective is yet to be shown. The work of Mackaness on the combination of cyclophosphamide

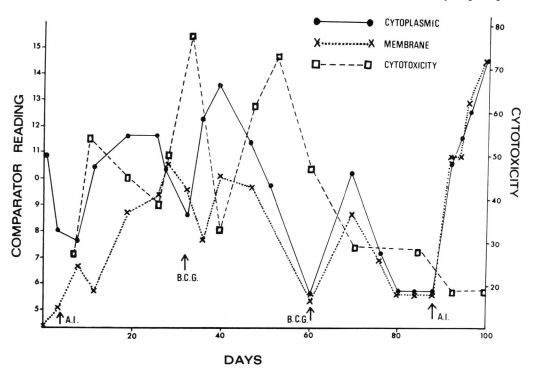

Fig. 10.22   Relationship between immune stimulation and production of antibodies and cytotoxic lymphocytes in a patient with malignant melanoma.

AI = auto-immunisation with autologous irradiated tumour cells.
BCG = oral administration of Bacillus Calmette-Guérin

Table 10.11   Immunotherapy of malignant melanoma

Specific—Active

Czajowski *et al.*	1967	Auto-immunisation with tumour cells plus rabbit immunoglobulin attached
Finney *et al.*	1969	Auto-immunisation with tumour homogenate
Van-Den Brenk	1969	Auto-immunisation with irradiated tumour cells
Lewis *et al.*	1969	Auto-immunisation with irradiated tumour cells
Ikonopisov *et al.*	1970	
Krementz *et al.*	1971	
Currie *et al.*	1971	
Seigler *et al.*	1972	Auto-immunisation with irradiated neuraminidase-treated cells
Simmons and Rios	1971	Neuraminidase-treated tumour cells plus BCG
Currie	1973	Auto-immunisation with irradiated tumour cells mixed with BCG
Gercovich	1974	Auto-immunisation in drainage of BCG scarification
Lewis *et al.*	1975	Auto-immunisation with irradiated tissue cultured cells plus oral BCG
Shibata *et al.*	1976	Auto-immunisation plus oral BCG

Table 10.12   Combined chemotherapy and immunotherapy of melanoma

Israel and Halpern	1972	Chemotherapy with an injection of *C. parvum*
Gutterman *et al.*	1974	DTIC and BCG
Ikonopisov	1975	
Gutterman *et al.*	1975b	
McCarthy and Milton	1975	
Currie and McElwaine	1975	DTIC—vincristine and auto-immunisation with irradiated tumour cells plus percutaneous BCG

and immunisation would strongly suggest that this might be a mechanism, and it therefore holds considerable hope for the future (Mackaness, Auclair and Lagrange, 1973).

CONCLUSIONS

It is clear that whatever method one uses in immunotherapy, the objectives should be clearly in one's mind. Is it to attempt to eradicate primary tumours, lymph node metastases, established metastases or to prevent the tumour progressing from one stage to the next? In this respect the important role of blood borne tumour cells must be a central consideration.

It has been appreciated for many years that tumour cells either singly or in clumps can survive passage through the circulation and ultimately give rise to widespread metastatic disease. This subject has been reviewed in recent years by one of the pioneers in this field (Wood, 1973).

The ability of such cells to survive the bloodstream and then adhere to and finally invade capillary walls is well established (Warren, 1973; Wood, 1958; Wood, 1964). This could well represent a critical 'weak spot' in the natural history of malignant tumours, and is worthy of close scrutiny from an immunological point of view, particularly when considering the role of antitumour antibodies and macrophages.

Simply to engage in a blind stimulation of the immune system, where derangement may be the major cause of failure in immune control, may be adding fuel to the fire and thereby will produce an even worse situation. Therefore, it is absolutely essential that we have some means of monitoring the effect of immune stimulation and relate these to changes in the growth or progression of measurable tumour or disease-free intervals after surgical excision.

An example of the relationship between some antitumour immune reactions and growth of lung metastases in a patient with melanoma can be seen in Figure 10.23. The relationship between antimembrane antibodies and appearance of metastases is seen in Figure 10.24.

In essence, what we need for the management of immunotherapy of malignancy is the equivalent of a blood sugar or serum electrolytes, to enable us to know when to advance and when to stop, and also when to alter a particular approach. It is likely that patients with melanoma as with other tumours are in every sense individuals and that at any moment in time the problem of tumour–host balance will be unique. Therefore, a unique approach may be needed in the manipulation of their immune system if this is to succeed in preventing metas-

tases and thus allow the other forms of therapy to be effective.

Malignant melanoma, with its wide spectrum of biological activity yet its potential for early diagnosis and well-defined states of progression, represents a model human tumour for such studies. Important lessons learned from this uncommon neoplasm will hopefully be applied to many other more frequent types of cancer.

COMMENT (G. W. M.)

Textbooks of medicine and surgery are often criticised because it is said that by the time they are published they are out of date. There is no

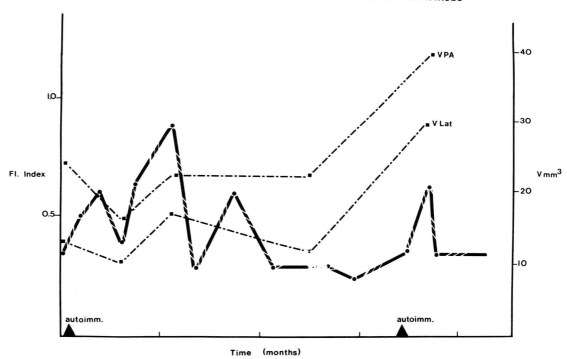

CORRELATION BETWEEN ANTI-MEMBRANE ANTIBODY AND SIZE OF METASTASES

Fig. 10.23   Relationship between size of lung metastases and alterations in antitumour immunity in a patient with malignant melanoma. Line with diagonal bars represents antitumour antibody levels as measured by fluorescence (FI) index.

VPA = measurement of volume of tumour by anteroposterior and lateral view X-rays of chest
VLAT = volume of lung metastases assessed by lateral X-ray film
Autoimm = immunisation with patient's own irradiated tumour cells

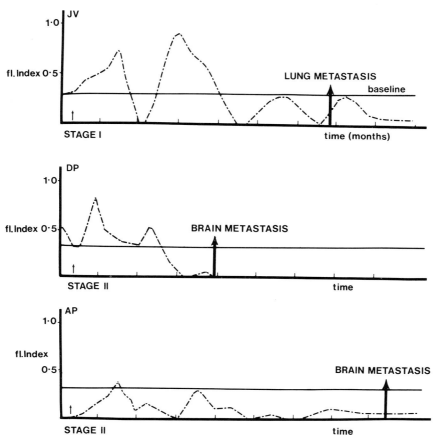

THE FALL OF ANTI-MEMBRANE ANTIBODY
PRIOR TO THE CLINICAL APPEARANCE OF METASTASIS

Fig. 10.24 Antimembrane antibody levels in three patients with melanoma tested sequentially; shows fall of antibody prior to clinical appearance of metastases. Dotted lines represent levels of antitumour antibody as measured by fluorescent indices in three individuals with malignant melanoma. (Proportion of tumour cells and controls demonstrating membrane immunofluorescence) (FI index)

field of medicine in which this could be more truthfully said at the present time than that of immunotherapy and the immunology of malignant disease. The very comprehensive review of Professor Lewis and his colleagues outlines the present status of the immunology of malignancy, but changes are taking place so rapidly that it would be impossible for this to remain a definitive statement for long.

From the clinicians' point of view immunotherapy of malignant melanoma often looks somewhat bewildering as there are so many trials currently taking place and the results seem to be confusing. I think it likely that within the course of the next few years immunotherapy for malignant melanoma will be developed to such a point that it will become a standard method of treatment, indeed there are already suggestions that this is the case with disease in which the prognosis is unfavourable. However, when new methods of therapy are introduced there is a danger that undue enthusiasm will lead to disappointment and the method fall into disrepute.

The present state of the 'game' as I see it, is as follows.

Patients subjected to immunotherapy may be divided into two groups:

1. Those who have local disease without proven generalised dissemination but in whom the prognosis is bad for reasons of the site or depth of penetration of the primary tumour or possible involvement of draining lymph nodes. In these patients the initial therapy is surgical, but immunotherapy may well prove useful as a means of inhibiting the establishment of generalised metastases. At the moment the most encouraging results appear to follow the use of BCG, but it may be a few years before the method is sufficiently established to become routine. Whether the effect of BCG will be enhanced by the use of chemotherapeutic agents such as DTIC is also not yet settled. As the matter is under discussion it is desirable that treatment with these techniques should, if possible, be carried out in special clinics where the results may be carefully assessed.

2. Patients with generalised dissemination usually have a short prognosis and consequently any method of therapy which may enhance their survival time and improve their health is desirable. Generally speaking most series report a small proportion of patients who respond to immune therapy. Although it is not yet proved in the scientific sense evidence so far available suggests that certain types of metastases will respond better than others. For example, the response to immunotherapy or chemotherapy for small metastases close to or in the skin is almost certainly better than the response of larger deposits in the lung, liver or brain. If metastases are very large, then the likelihood of response is much less whatever the method of treatment used. Accordingly, to reiterate as has already been stated elsewhere in this book the follow-up of patients with malignant melanoma is of vital importance as far as treatment is concerned if metastatic disease is to be recognised at the earliest possible moment. Metastases in the liver probably respond worse to all forms of therapy than those at any other site. An intermediate site where transient improvement is often achieved

by chemotherapy, less so with immunotherapy, are metastases in the lung provided they are few and small. Metastases in the brain do not respond to immunotherapy, and it also frequently happens that patients who have metastatic disease in other sites, which respond initially to immunotherapy, will come back in less than two years with cerebral metastases.

We have also shown in figures quoted elsewhere in this book that metastases in the brain occasionally respond with a transient benefit with several forms of chemotherapy, notably DTIC, and also with a combination of chemotherapy and radiotherapy. However, the response is unlikely to be permanent, except in the very rare case of a resectable solitary cerebral metastasis.

Finally, the methods of measuring immunological competence are at an interesting stage of development, but unfortunately the immunological assessment in an individual patient is difficult and it is also difficult to be certain of the validity of the various measurements in relation to the behaviour of the tumour in any individual case. It is in this field that we are likely to have advances more rapidly than in others. One of the reasons why there is such difficulty in obtaining unified and easily interpretable results is probably that the balance between the host and the tumour is not constant but is likely to undergo variation quite rapidly, and this variation may be tissue specific. I have already mentioned that metastases in the brain will frequently occur when those at other sites have apparently been satisfactorily treated with chemotherapy or immunotherapy and that metastases in the liver fail to respond to both. Accordingly, the number of 'moving parts' in this problem is immense because not only is the patient as a whole to be assessed but it may well be that the relationship between tumour deposits in his separate tissues are also different from one another. The difficulty is made worse by the fact, as Professor Lewis mentions, that animal models and tissue culture models, although interesting in the biological way, may not be precise tools when one wishes to measure results against the behaviour of a tumour in man.

REFERENCES

Alexander, P. (1972) Foetal antigens in cancer. *Nature (Lond.)*, **235**, 137.

Alexander, P., Bensted, J. & Delorme, E. J. (1967) Cellular immune response to primary sarcomata in rats. II. Abnormal response of nodes draining. *Proceedings of the Royal Society of London* (B), **174**, 237.

Allen, A. C. & Spitz, S. (1953) Malignant melanoma: a clinicopathological analysis of the criteria for prognosis and diagnosis. *Cancer*, **6**, 1.

Ambus, U., Mavligit, G. M., Gutterman, J. U., *et al.* (1974) Specific and non-specific immunologic reactivity of regional lymph nodes lymphocytes in human malignancy. *International Journal of Cancer*, **14**, 291.

Amery, W. K. (1976) Double-blind levamisole trial in resectable lung cancer. *Annals of the New York Academy of Sciences* (in press).

Anderson, N. G. & Coggin, J. H. (1972) Embryonic antigens in virally transformed cells. In *Membranes and Viruses in Immunopathology*, ed. Good, R. A. & Day, S. B., p. 217. New York: Academic Press.

Avis, P. J. G. & Lewis, M. G. (1973) Tumour associated foetal antigens in human tumours. *Journal of the National Cancer Institute*, **51**, 1063.

Bailly, C. (1972) L'histoprogostic du mélanoma malin cutané. Thesis. *Associalia Corporature des Etudiants en Médecine de Lyon*. Lyon.

Baker, M. A. & Taub, R. N. (1973a) BCG in malignant melanoma. *Lancet*, i, 1117.

Baker, M. A. & Taub, R. N. (1973b) Immunotherapy of human cancer. *Progress in Allergy*, **17**, 227.

Baldwin, R. W. (1955) Immunity to methylcholanthrene-induced tumours in inbred rats following atrophy and regression of the implanted tumours. *British Journal of Cancer*, **9**, 652.

Baldwin, R. W., Embleton, M. J., Price, M. R., *et al.* (1974a) Immunity in the tumour-bearing host and its modification by serum factors. *Cancer*, **34**, 1452.

Baldwin, R. W., Glaves, D. & Vose, B. M. (1974b) Immunogenicity of embryonic antigens associated with chemically induced rat tumours. *International Journal of Cancer*, **13**, 135.

Baldwin, R. W., Price, M. R. & Robins, R. A. (1972) Blocking of lymphocyte-mediated cytotoxicity for rat hepatoma cells by tumour-specific antigen–antibody complexes. *Nature (New Biology)*, **238**, 185.

Belisario, J. C. & Milton, G. W. (1961) The experimental local therapy of cutaneous metastases of malignant melanoblastomas with cow pox vaccine or colcemid (demecolcine or omaine). *Australian Journal of Dermatology*, **6**, 113.

Birkmayer, G. D., Balda, B. R. & Miller, F. (1974) Oncorna-viral information in human melanoma. *European Journal of Cancer*, **10**, 419.

Birkmayer, G. D., Hammer, C., Eberhard, H. D., *et al.* (1975) A tumour-specific antigen associated with reverse transcriptase in human melanoma. *Behring Institute Mitteilungen*, **56**, 107.

Bloom, E. T., Ossorio, R. C. & Brosman, S. A. (1974) Cell-mediated cytotoxicity against bladder cancer. *International Journal of Cancer*, **14**, 326.

Blumming, A. Z., Vogel, C. L. & Ziegler, J. L. (1972) Immunological effects of BCG in malignant melanoma. Two modes of administration compared. *Annals of Internal Medicine*, **76**, 405.

Blumming, A. Z., Vogel, C. L. Ziegler, J. L., *et al.* (1972) Delayed cutaneous sensitivity reactions to extracts of autologous malignant melanoma—a second look. *Journal of the National Cancer Institute*, **48**, 17.

Bodenham, D. C. (1968) A study of 650 observed malignant melanomas in the South-West region. *Annals of the Royal College of Surgeons of England*, **43**, 218.

Bodurtha, A. J., Chee, D. O., Laucius, J. F., *et al.* (1975) Clinical and immunological significance of human melanoma cytotoxic antibody. *Cancer Research*, **35**, 189.

Bourgoin, J. J., Vitris, M., Rifa, J., *et al.* (1975) Study of peripheral human lymphocytes forming spontaneous rosettes with sheep erythrocytes in malignant melanoma. *Behring Institute Mitteilungen*, **56**, 263.

Brandes, L. J., Galton, D. A. G. & Wiltshaw, E. (1971) New approach to immunotherapy of melanoma. *Lancet*, ii, 293.

Brawn, R. J. (1971) *In vitro* desensitisation of sensitised murine lymphocytes by a serum factor (soluble antigen?). *Proceedings of the National Academy of Sciences, Washington*, **68**, 1634.

Burdick, K. H. (1960) Malignant melanoma treated with vaccinia infections. *Archives of Dermatology*, **82**, 438.

Burdick, K. H. & Hawk, W. A. (1964) Vitiligo in a case of vaccinia virus treated melanoma. *Cancer*, **17**, 708.

Burg, G. & Braun-Falco, O. (1972) The cellular stromal reaction in malignant melanoma. A cyto-chemical investigation. *Archiv für Dermatologische Forschung*, **245**, 318.

Butterworth, C., Oon, C. J., Westbury, G., *et al.* (1974) T-lymphocyte responses in patients with malignant melanoma. *European Journal of Cancer*, **10**, 639.

Byrne, M., Heppner, G., Stolbach, L., *et al.* (1973) Tumour immunity in melanoma patients assessed by colony inhibition and microcytotoxicity methods: a preliminary report. *National Cancer Institute Monographs*, **37**, 3.

Canevari, S., Fossati, G., Della Porta, G., *et al.* (1975) Humoral cytoxicity in melanoma patients and its correlation with the extent and the course of the disease. *International Journal of Cancer*, **16**, 72.

Cano, P., Jerry, L. M., Lewis, M. G., *et al.* (1976) Immune complexes in the serum of patients with malignancy. (Paper in preparation.)

Carrel, S. & Theilkaes, L. (1973) Evidence for a tumour-associated antigen in human malignant melanoma. *Nature (Lond.)*, **242**, 609.

Césarini, J. P., Bonneau, H. & Calas, E. (1968) Le halo-naevus (Naevus de Sutton). *Annals de Dermatologie et Syphiligraphie*, **95**, 505.

Char, D. H., Hollinshead, A. C., Cogan, D. G., et al. (1974) Cutaneous delayed hypersensitivity reactions to soluble melanoma antigen in patients with ocular melanoma. *New England Journal of Medicine*, **291**, 274.

Claudy, A. J., Kac, J., Pelletier, N., et al. (1975) Prognostic correlations in malignant melanoma. *European Journal of Cancer*, **11**, 821.

Cochran, A. J. (1969) Malignant melanoma: a review of 10 years' experience in Glasgow, Scotland. *Cancer*, **23**, 1190.

Cochran, A. J., Jehn, V. W. & Gothoska, B. P. (1972) Cell-mediated immunity to malignant melanoma. *Lancet*, i, 1340.

Cochran, A. J., Mackie, R. M., Thomas, C. E., et al. (1973) Cellular immunity to breast carcinomas and malignant melanoma. *British Journal of Cancer*, **28**, 77.

Cochran, A. J., Ross, C. E., Mackie, R. M., et al. (1975) The immune status of patients with malignant melanoma. *Behring Institute Mitteilungen*, **56**, 125.

Cochran, A. J., Spilg, W. G. S., Mackie, R. M., et al. (1972) Post-operative depression of tumour-directed cell-mediated immunity in patients with malignant disease. *British Medical Journal*, iv, 67.

Cochran, A. J., Thomas, C. E., Spilg, W. G. S., et al. (1973) Tumour-directed cellular immunity in malignant melanoma and its modification by surgical treatment. *Yale Journal of Biology and Medicine*, **46**, 650.

Coggin, J. H. & Anderson, N. G. (1974) Embryonic antigens: some central problems. *Advances in Cancer Research*, **19**, 105.

Coley, W. B. (1893) Treatment of malignant tumours by repeated inoculations of erysipelas with a report of 10 cases. *Medical Record* (N.Y.), **43**, 60.

Coley, W. B. & Hoguet, J. P. (1916) Melanotic cancer. *Annals of Surgery*, **64**, 206.

Coons, A. H., Creech, H. J. & Jones, R. N. (1941) Immunological properties of an antibody containing a fluorescent group. *Proceedings of the Society of Experimental Biology and Medicine*, **47**, 200.

Cooper, H. L. (1970) Lymphocyte stimulation in malignant melanoma. *New England Journal of Medicine*, **283**, 369.

Copeman, P. W. M., Lewis, M. G., Phillips, T. M., et al. (1973) Immunological associations of the halo naevus with cutaneous malignant melanoma. *British Journal of Dermatology*, **88**, 127.

Couperous, M. & Rucker, R. C. (1954) Histopathological diagnosis of malignant melanoma. *Medical Journal of Australia*, **2**, 1028.

Currie, G. A. (1972) 80 years of immunotherapy. *British Journal of Cancer*, **26**, 141.

Currie, G. A. (1973) Effects of active immunization with irradiated tumour cells on specific serum inhibitors of cell mediated immunity in patients with disseminated cancer. *British Journal of Cancer*, **28**, 25.

Currie, G. A. & Bagshawe, K. D. (1967) The masking of antigens on trophoblasts and tumour cells. *Lancet*, i, 708.

Currie, G. A. & Basham, C. (1972) Serum mediated inhibition of the immunological reactions of the patient to his own tumour: A possible role for circulating antigen. *British Journal of Cancer*, **26**, 427.

Currie, G. A., Lejeune, F. & Hamilton-Fairley, G. (1971) Immunisation with irradiated tumour cells and specific cytotoxicity in malignant melanoma. *British Medical Journal*, **2**, 305.

Currie, G. A. & McElwain, T. J. (1975) Active immunotherapy as an adjunct to chemotherapy in the treatment of disseminated malignant melanoma: a pilot study. *British Journal of Cancer*, **31**, 143.

Curtis, J. E. (1971) Adoptive immunotherapy in the treatment of advanced malignant melanoma. *Proceedings of the American Association for Cancer Research*, **12**, 52.

Czajowski, N. P., Rosenblatt, M., Wolf, P. L., et al. (1967) A new method for active immunization to autologous human tumour tissue. *Lancet*, ii, 905.

Das Gupta, T., Bowden, L. & Berg, T. W. (1963) Malignant melanoma of unknown primary origin. *Surgery, Gynecology and Obstetrics*, **117**, 341.

Davignon, L., Lemonde, P., Robillard, P., et al. (1970) BCG vaccination and leukaemia mortality. *Lancet*, ii, 638.

Decker, P. J. & Pilch, Y. H., (1972) Mediation of immunity to tumour-specific transplantation antigens by RNA inhibition of isograft growth in rats. *Cancer Research*, **32**, 839.

De Gast, G. C., The, T. H., Schraffordt-Koops, H., et al., (1975) Humoral and cell-mediated immune response in patients with malignant melanoma. I. In-vitro lymphocyte reactivity to PHA and antigens following immunization. *Cancer*, **36**, 1289.

Della Porta, G., Fossati, G. & Canevari, S. (1973) Complement-dependent cytotoxicity of serum of patients with malignant melanoma. *Proceedings of the American Association for Cancer Research*, **14**, 33.

De Vries, J. E., Cornain, S. & Rümke, P. (1975) Humoral and cellular immunity in melanoma patients. *Behring Institute Mitteilungen*, **56**, 148.

De Vries, J. E., Rümke, P. & Bernheim, J. L. (1972) Cytotoxic lymphocytes in melanoma patients. *International Journal of Cancer*, **9**, 567.

Diluzio, N. R., McNamee, R., Olcay, A., et al. (1974) Inhibition of tumour growth by recognition factor. *Proceedings of the Society of Experimental Biology and Medicine*, **145**, 311.

Eberman, A. A. (1896) Beitrag zur Casuistik der melanotischen Geschwulste. *Deutsche Zeitschrift für Chirurgie*, **43**, 498.

Ebner, H. Von & Niebauer, G. (1968) Elektronenoptische Befunde zum Pigmentverlust heim Naevus Sutton. *Dermatologica*, **137**, 345.

Embleton, M. J. & Price, M. R. (1975) Inhibition of in-vitro lymphocytotoxicity reactions against tumour cells by melanoma membrane extracts. *Behring Institute Mitteilungen*, **56**, 157.

Epstein, W. L., Sagebeil, R., Spitler, L., *et al.* (1973) Halo naevi and melanoma. *Journal of the American Medical Association*, **225**, 373.

Evans, R. & Alexander, P. (1972) Role of macrophages in tumour immunity. *Immunology*, **23**, 615.

Eve, F. (1903) Lecture on melanoma. *London Practitioner*, p. 165.

Everall, J. D., O'Doherty, E. J., Wand, J., *et al.* (1975) Treatment of primary melanoma by intralesional vaccinia before excision. *Lancet*, ii, 583.

Everson, J. C. & Cole, W. H. (1966) *Spontaneous Regression of Cancer*. London: Saunders.

Falk, R. E., Mann, P. & Langen, B. (1973) Cell-mediated immunity to human tumors. *Archives of Surgery*, **107**, 261.

Fass, L., Herberman, R. B., Ziegler, J. L., *et al.* (1970) Cutaneous hypersensitivity reactions to autologous extracts of malignant melanoma cells. *Lancet*, i, 166.

Federman, J. L., Lewis, M. G. & Clarke, W. H. (1974) Tumor-associated antibodies to ocular and cutaneous melanoma: negative interaction with normal choroidal melanocytes. *Journal of the National Cancer Institute*, **52**, 587.

Federman, J. L., Lewis, M. G., Clarke, W. H., *et al.* (1974) Tumor-associated antibodies in the serum of ocular melanoma patients. *Transactions; American Academy of Ophthalmology and Otolaryngology*, **78**, 784.

Findlay, G. H. (1957) The histology of Sutton's naevus. *British Journal of Dermatology*, **69**, 389.

Finney, J. W., Byers, E. H. & Wilson, R. H. (1969) Studies on tumour immunity. *Cancer Research*, **20**, 351.

Fishman, M. (1961) Antibody formation *in vitro*. *Journal of Experimental Medicine*, **114**, 837.

Foley, E. J. (1953) Antigenic properties of methylcholanthrene-induced tumours in mice in the strain of origin. *Cancer Research*, **13**, 835.

Fossati, G., Colnaghi, M. E., Della Porta, G., *et al.* (1971) Cellular and humoral immunity against human malignant melanoma. *International Journal of Cancer*, **8**, 344.

Frenster, J. H. & Rogoway, W. M. (1970) Clinical use of activated autologous lymphocytes for human cancer immunity. In 'Oncology'—Yearbooks in Medicine, ed. Cumley, R. W. & McKay, J. E., p. 327. Chicago: Year Book Medical Publishers.

Gauci, C. L. (1975) The macrophage content of human malignant melanomas. *Behring Institute Mitteilungen*, **56**, 73.

Gauthier, Y., Surleve-Bazeille, J. E., Gauthier, O., *et al.* (1975) Ultrastructure of halo naevi. *Journal of Cutaneous Pathology*, **3**, 71.

Gercovich, F. G. (1974) Active specific immunization in malignant melanoma. *Medical Journal of Pediatric Oncology* (in press).

Ghose, T., Norvell, W. T., Guclu, A., *et al.* (1972) Immunotherapy of cancer with chlorambucil-carrying antibody. *British Medical Journal*, iii, 495.

Ghose, T., Norvell, S. T., Guclu, A., *et al.* (1975) Immunochemotherapy of human malignant melanoma with chlorambucil-carrying antibody. *European Journal of Cancer*, **11**, 321.

Gold, P. & Freedman, S. (1965) Demonstration of tumour-specific antigens in human colonic carcinomata by immunological tolerance and absorption techniques. *Journal of Experimental Medicine*, **121**, 439.

Goldman M. (1960) Antigenic analysis of *Entamoeba histolytica* by means of fluorescent antibody. I. instrumentation for microfluorimetry of stained amoebae. *Experimental Parasitology*, **9**, 25.

Goldman, M. (1967) An improved microfluorimeter for measuring brightness of fluorescent antibody reactions. *Journal of Histochemistry and Cytochemistry*, **15**, 38.

Goldman, M. (1968) *Fluorescent Antibody Methods*. New York: Academic Press.

Golub, S. H. & Morton, D. L. (1974) Sensitization of lymphocytes in vitro against human melanoma-associated antigens. *Nature (Lond.)*, **251**, 161.

Goodier, D. P., Horning, M. O., Leong, S. P. L., *et al.* (1972) Immune responses induced by human malignant melanoma in the rabbit. *Surgery*, **72**, 737.

Gorodilova, V. V. & Hollinshead, A. (1975) Melanoma antigens that produce cell-mediated immune responses in melanoma patients: Joint U.S.–U.S.S.R. study. *Science, N.Y.*, **190**, 391.

Grant, R. M., Mackie, R. M., Cochran, A. J., *et al.* (1974) Results of administering BCG to patients with melanoma. *Lancet*, ii, 1096.

Gray, B. K., Mehigan, J. T. & Morton, D. L. (1971) Demonstration of antibody in melanoma patients cytotoxic to human melanoma cells. *Proceedings of the American Association for Cancer Research*, **12**, 79.

Grosser, N. & Thompson, D. M. P. (1975) Cell-mediated antitumour immunity in breast cancer patients evaluated by antigen-induced leukocyte adherence inhibition in test tubes. *Cancer Research*, **35**, 2571.

Gupta, R. K. & Morton, D. L. (1975) Suggestive evidence for *in vivo* binding of specific antitumour antibodies of human melanomas. *Cancer Research*, **35**, 58.

Gutterman, J. U., Mavligit, G., McBride, C., *et al.* (1973a) Active immunotherapy with BCG for recurrent malignant melanoma. *Lancet*, i, 1208.

Gutterman, J. U., Mavligit, G. M., McBride, C., *et al.* (1973b) BCG stimulation of immune responsiveness in patients with malignant melanoma. Preliminary report. *Cancer*, **32**, 321.

Gutterman, J. U., Mavligit, G., Reed, R. C., *et al.* (1974) Immunochemotherapy of human cancer. *Seminars in Oncology*, **1**, 409.

Gutterman, J. U., Mavligit, G., Reed, R. C., *et al.* (1975a) Immunology and immunotherapy of human malignant melanoma: historical review and perspectives for the future. *Seminars in Oncology*, **2**, 155.

Gutterman, J. U., Mavligit, G., Reed, R. C., *et al.* (1975b) Adjuvant immunotherapy with BCG for recurrent malignant melanoma. *Behring Institute Mitteilungen*, **56**, 199.

Halliday, W. J., Maluish, A. & Isibister, W. H. (1974) Detection of anti-tumour cell-mediated immunity and serum blocking factors in cancer patients by the Leucocyte Adherence Inhibition test. *British Journal of Cancer*, **29**, 31.

Halliday, W. J. & Miller, S. (1972) Leucocyte adherence inhibition: a simple test for cell mediated immunity and serum blocking factors. *International Journal of Cancer*, **9**, 477.

Halpern, B. N., Biozzi, G., Stiffel, C., *et al.* (1959) Effect de la stimulation du système réticulo-endothélial par l'inoculation du bacille de Calmette-Guérin sur la développement l'epithelioma atypique T-8 de Guérin chez le rat. *Comptes Rendus des Séances de la Société de Biologie et de ses Filiales* (Paris), **153**, 919.

Hamilton-Fairly, G. (1969) Immunity to malignant disease in man. *British Medical Journal*, ii, 467.

Handley, W. S. (1907) The pathology of melanotic growths. *Lancet*, i, 927.

Hartmann, D. P. & Lewis, M. G. (1974) Presence and possible role of anti-IgG antibodies in human malignancy. *Lancet*, i, 1318.

Hartmann, D. P., Lewis, M. G., Proctor, J. W., *et al.* (1974) *In-vitro* interactions between antitumour antibodies and anti-antibodies in malignancy. *Lancet*, ii, 1481.

Haskill, J. S. (1973) A micro-colony-inhibition method for quantitation for tumour immunity. *Journal of the National Cancer Institute*, **51**, 1581.

Haskill, J. S. & Raymond, M. S. (1973) New method for the rapid quantitation of immunofluorescence. *Journal of the National Cancer Institute*, **51**, 159.

Hellström, I. (1967) Colony inhibition technique for the demonstration of tumour cell destruction by lymphoid cells *in vitro*. *International Journal of Cancer*, **2**, 65.

Hellström, I., Hellström, K. E., Bill, A. N., *et al.* (1969) Demonstration of cell bound and humoral immunity against neuroblastoma cells. *Proceedings of the National Academy of Sciences*, Washington, **60**, 1231.

Hellström, I., Hellström, K. E., Sjögren, H. O., *et al.* (1971) Demonstration of cell-mediated immunity in human neoplasms of various histological types. *International Journal of Cancer*, **1**, 1.

Hellström, I., Hellström, K. E., Sjögren, H. O., *et al.* (1973) Destruction of cultivated melanoma cells by lymphocytes from healthy black (North American Negro) donors. *International Journal of Cancer*, **11**, 116.

Hellström, I., Sjögren, H. O., Warner, G. A., *et al.* (1971) Blocking of cell-mediated tumour immunity by sera from patients with growing neoplasms. *International Journal of Cancer*, **1**, 226.

Hellstöm, I., Warner, G. A., Hellström, K. E., *et al.* (1973) Sequential studies on cell-mediated tumour immunity and blocking serum activity in 10 patients with malignant melanoma. *International Journal of Cancer*, **11**, 280.

Heppner, G., Henry, E., Stolbach, L., *et al.* (1975) Problems in the clinical use of the microcytotoxicity assay for measuring cell-mediated immunity to tumour cells. *Cancer Research*, **35**, 1931.

Heppner, G. H., Stolbach, L., Byrne, M., *et al.* (1973) Cell-mediated reactivity to tumour antigens in patients with malignant melanoma. *International Journal of Cancer*, **11**, 240.

Herberman, R. B., Hollinshead, A. C., Char, D., *et al.* (1975) *In-vivo* and *in-vitro* studies of cell-mediated immune response to antigens associated with malignant melanoma. *Behring Institute Mitteilungen*, **56**, 131.

Hersey, P. (1975) Personal communication.

Hersey, P., MacLennon, I. C. M. & Campbell, A. C. (1973) Cytotoxicity against human leukemic cells. I. Demonstration of antibody-dependent lymphocyte killing of human allogeneic myeloblasts. *Clinical and Experimental Immunology*, **14**, 159.

Hersh, E. M., Gutman, J. U., Mavligit, G. M., *et al.* (1975) Approaches to the study of tumour antigens and tumour immunity in malignant melanoma. *Behring Institute Mitteilungen*, **56**, 139.

Hibbs, J. B. (1973) Macrophage non-immunologic recognition; target cell factors related to contact inhibition. *Science* (N.Y.), **180**, 868.

Hibbs, J. B., Lambert, L. H. & Remington, J. S. (1972) Possible role of macrophage-mediated non-specific cytotoxicity in tumour resistance. *Nature (New Biology)*, **235**, 48.

Himmelweitt, F. (1957) *The Collected Papers of Paul Ehrlich*, Vol. II, p. 178. London: Pergamon Press.

Holborow, E. J. (1970) *Standardization in Immunofluorescence*. Oxford: Blackwell.

Hollinshead, A. C. (1975) Analysis of soluble melanoma cell membrane antigens in metastatic cells from various organs and further studies of antigens present in primary melanoma. *Cancer*, **36**, 1282.

Hollinshead, A. C., Herberman, R. B., Jaffurs, W. T., *et al.* (1974) Soluble antigens of human malignant melanoma cells. *Cancer*, **23**, 1235.

Horn, L. & Horn, H. L. (1971) An immunological approach to the therapy of cancer. *Lancet*, ii, 466.

Hughes, L. E. & Lytton, B. (1964) Antigenic properties of human tumours; delayed cutaneous hypersensitivity reactions. *British Medical Journal*, i, 209.

Humble, J. G., Jayne, W. H. W. & Pulvertaft, R. J. V. (1956) Biological interactions between lymphocytes and other cells. *British Journal of Haematology*, **2**, 283.

Humphrey, L. J., Lincoln, P. M. & Griffen, W. O. (1968) Immunologic response in patients with disseminated cancer. *Annals of Surgery*, **168**, 374.

Hunter-Craig, I. D., Newton, K. A., Westbury, G., et al. (1970) Use of vaccinia virus in the treatment of metastatic malignant melanoma. *British Medical Journal*, ii, 512.

Ikonopisov, R. L. (1975) The use of BCG in the combined treatment of malignant melanoma. *Behring Institute Mitteilungen*, **56**, 206.

Ikonopisov, R. L., Lewis, M. G., Hunter-Craig, I. D., et al. (1970) Autoimmunization with irradiated tumour cells in human malignant melanoma. *British Medical Journal*, ii, 752.

Israel, L. & Edelstein, R. (1973) Non-specific immunostimulation with *Corynebacterium parvum* in human cancer. *Twenty-sixth Annual M. D. Anderson Symposium*. Baltimore: Williams and Wilkins.

Israel, L. & Halpern, B. (1972) Le *Corynebacterium parvum* dans les cancer advancés. Première évaluation de practivité thérapeutique de celle immunostimulien. *Nouvelle Presse Medicale*, **1**, 19.

Iverson, O. H., Larsen, T. E., Grude, T. H., et al. (1976) Histological classification of malignant melanoma in relation to prognosis and cytogenesis. *Excerpta Medica* (in press).

Jacobs, J. B., Edelstein, L. M., Synder, L. M., et al. (1975) Ultrastructural evidence for destruction in the halo naevus. *Cancer Research*, **35**, 352.

Jehn, D., Nathanson, L. & Schwartz, R. S. (1970) *In-vitro* lymphocyte stimulation by a soluble tumour antigen in malignant melanoma. *New England Journal of Medicine*, **283**, 329.

Jerne, N. K. (1974) In *Cellular Selection and Regulation in Immune Response*, ed. Edelman, G. M., p. 39. New York: Raven Press.

Jerry, L. M., Adams, L. S., Sladowski, J. P., et al. (1976) Direct detection of immune complexes in sera of patients with malignant melanoma. *European Journal of Cancer* (submitted for publication).

Johansson, B. & Ljungovist, A. (1974) Localization of immunoglobulins in urinary bladder tumours. *Acta pathologica et microbiologica scandinavica (A)*, **82**, 559.

Jones, J. M. & Feldman, D. (1975) Immunogenic and antigenic properties of a rat Maloney sarcoma. *Behring Institute Mitteilungen*, **56**, 14.

Kaliss, N. (1958) Immunological enhancement of tumour homografts in mice. A review. *Cancer Research*, **18**, 992.

Kanner, S. P., Mardiney, M. R. & Mairgi, R. J. (1970) Experience with a mixed lymphocyte tumour reaction as a method of detecting antigenic differences between normal and neoplastic cells. *Journal of Immunology*, **105**, 1052.

Katz, A. & Digby, J. W. (1965) Malignant melanoma and dermatomyositis. *Canadian Medical Association Journal*, **93**, 1367.

Keller, R. (1973) Evidence for compromise of tumour immunity in rats by non-specific serum factor that inactivates macrophages. *British Journal of Experimental Pathology*, **54**, 298.

Klein, E. (1969) Hypersensitivity reaction at tumour site. *Cancer Research*, **29**, 2351.

Klein, E. & Holterman, O. A. (1972) Immunotherapeutic approaches to the management of neoplasms. *National Cancer Institute Monographs*, **35**, 379.

Klein, E., Holterman, O. A., Helm, F., et al. (1975) Immunologic approaches to the management of primary and secondary tumours involving the skin and soft tissues. Review of a ten year programme. *Transplantation Proceedings*, **7**, 927.

Klein, E., Holterman, O. A., Papermaster, et al. (1973) Immunologic approaches in various types of cancer with the use of BCG and PPD. *National Cancer Institute Monographs*, **39**, 229.

Klein, G., Clifford, P., Klein, E., et al. (1966) Search for tumour specific immune reactions in Burkitt's Lymphoma patients by the membrane immunofluorescence reaction. *Proceedings of the National Academy of Sciences of the United States of America*, **55**, 1628.

Kopf, A. W. (1971) Host defences against malignant melanoma. *Hospital Practice*, Oct., 116.

Kopf, A. W., Morrill, S. D. & Silberg, I. (1965) Broad spectrum of leukoderm acquisitum centrifugum. *Archives of Dermatology*, **92**, 14.

Krementz, E. T., Samuals, M. S., Wallace, J. H., et al. (1971) Clinical experience in immunotherapy of cancer. *Surgery, Gynecology and Obstetrics*, **133**, 209.

Lancet (1975) Non-renal neoplasms and the kidney. *Lancet*, i, 24.

Landazuri, M. O. de, Kedar, E. & Fahey, J. L. (1975) Synergism between cytotoxic cells and immune serum in a syngeneic lymphoma: characterization of two types of cytotoxic cells. *Behring Institute Mitteilungen*, **56**, 3.

Lawrence, H. S. (1963) Transfer factor. *Advances in Immunology*, **11**, 95.

Lejeune, F. J. (1973) Harding–Passey melanoma in the Balb/C mouse as a model for studying the interaction between host macrophages and tumour cells. *Yale Journal of Biology and Medicine*, **46**, 368.

Lejeune, F. J. (1975) Role of macrophages in immunity, with special reference to tumour immunology. A review. *Biomedicine*, **22**, 25.

Levi, E. (1963) Preparation of an antiserum specific to a spontaneous mouse leukemia after the induction of artificial immunological tolerance to normal mouse tissue. *Nature (Lond.)*, **199**, 501.

Lewis, M. G. (1967a) Malignant melanoma in Uganda: the relationship between pigmentation and malignant melanoma on the soles of the feet. *British Journal of Cancer*, **21**, 483.

Lewis, M. G. (1967b) Possible immunological factors in human malignant melanoma in Uganda. *Lancet*, ii, 921.

Lewis, M. G. (1971) Host factors in human malignant melanoma. In *Pathology Annual*, ed. Sommers, S. Vol. 6, p. 171. New York: Appleton-Century-Crofts.

Lewis, M. G. (1972) Circulating humoral antibodies in cancer. *Medical Clinics of North America*, **56**, 481.

Lewis, M. G. (1973a) Tumour-specific antigens in melanoma. In *Seventh National Cancer Conference Proceedings*, p. 77. Philadelphia: Lippincott.

Lewis, M. G. (1973b) Mechanisms of humoral tumor immunity in malignant melanoma. In *Proceedings of the Tenth Canadian Cancer Research Conference*, ed. Scholefield, P. G., p. 113. University of Toronto Press.

Lewis, M. G. (1974a) Technical and interpretative problems with immunofluorescence. In *Recent Results in Cancer Research*, ed. Mathé, G. & Weiner, R. Vol. 45, p. 58. Berlin: Springer-Verlag.

Lewis, M. G. (1974b) Immunology and the melanomas. *Current Topics in Microbiology and Immunology*, **63**, 49.

Lewis, M. G. & Copeman, P. W. M. (1972) Halo naevus—a frustrated malignant melanoma. *British Medical Journal*, ii, 47.

Lewis, M. G. & Kiryabwire, J. W. M. (1968) Malignant melanoma in Uganda—aspects of behaviour and natural history. *Cancer*, **21**, 876.

Lewis, M. G. & Phillips, T. M. (1972a) The specificity of surface membrane immunofluorescence in human malignant melanoma. *International Journal of Cancer*, **10**, 105.

Lewis, M. G. & Phillips, T. M. (1972b) Separation of two distinct tumour associated antibodies in the serum of melanoma patients. *Journal of the National Cancer Institute*, **49**, 915.

Lewis, M. G. & Raymond, M. J. (1975) Humoral and cellular host reactions to melanoma antigens. *Behring Institute Mitteilungen*, **56**, 120.

Lewis, M. G. & Sheikh, M. A. (1975) Evidence for tumour specific antigens in human malignant melanoma. *Behring Institute Mitteilungen*, **56**, 78.

Lewis, M. G., Hartmann, D. P. & Jerry, L. M. (1976) Antibodies and anti-antibodies in malignancy. *Annals of the New York Academy of Sciences* (in press).

Lewis, M. G., Jerry, L. M. & Shibata, H. (1975) Prospectives for immunotherapy of malignant melanoma. *Excerpta Medica* (in press).

Lewis, M. G., Loughridge, L. W. & Phillips, T. M. (1971) Immunological studies on a patient with the nephrotic syndrome associated with malignancy of non-renal origin. *Lancet*, ii, 134.

Lewis, M. G., McCloy, E. & Blake, J. (1973) The significance of circulating antibody in the localization of human malignant melanoma. *British Journal of Surgery*, **60**, 443.

Lewis, M. G., Rowden, G. & Burke, B. (1976) Immune reactions in patients with malignant melanoma and possible causes of failure of control. *Excerpta Medica* (in press).

Lewis, M. G., Avis, P. J. G., Phillips, T. M., *et al.* (1973) Tumour specific and tumour associated antigens in human malignant melanoma. *Yale Journal of Biology and Medicine*, **46**, 661.

Lewis, M. G., Humble, J. G., Lee, E. S., *et al.* (1971) The effects of intravenous phytohaemagglutinin in a patient with disseminated malignant melanoma: a clinical and immunological study. *Revue européene d'études cliniques et biologiques*, **16**, 924.

Lewis, M. G., Ikonopisov, R. L., Nairn, R. C., *et al.* (1969) Tumour specific antibodies in human malignant melanoma and their relationship to the extent of the disease. *British Medical Journal*, ii, 547.

Lewis, M. G., Mansell, P. W. A., Jerry, L. M., *et al.* (1976) Individual specific antigens on the surface of the human malignant melanoma cells (in preparation).

Lewis, M. G., Phillips, T. M., Cook, K. B., *et al.* (1971) Possible explanation for the loss of detectable antibody in patients with disseminated malignant melanoma. *Nature (Lond.)*, **232**, 52.

Lewis, M. G., Proctor, J. W., Thomson, D. M. P., *et al.* (1976) Cellular localization of immunoglobulin within human malignant melanomas. *British Journal of Cancer* (in press).

Lieberman, R., Epstein, W. L. & Fudenberg, H. H. (1974) Immunopathologic changes in patients with cutaneous malignant melanoma following intradermal inoculation of BCG. Correlation with cell-mediated immunity. *International Journal of Cancer*, **14**, 401.

Lieberman, R., Wybran, J. & Epstein, W. L. (1975) The immunologic and histopathologic changes of BCG mediated tumour regression in patients with malignant melanoma. *Cancer*, **35**, 756.

Little, J. H. (1972) Histology and prognosis in cutaneous malignant melanoma. In *Melanoma and Skin Cancer. Proceedings of the International Cancer Conference, Sydney, N.S.W.*, p. 107. Sydney: Government Printer.

Loughridge, L. W. & Lewis, M. G. (1971) Nephrotic syndrome in malignant disease of non-renal origin. *Lancet*, i, 256.

McBride, W. H., Jones, J. & Weir, D. M. (1975) Target cell killing by *C. parvum* stimulated cells. *Behring Institute Mitteilungen*, **56**, 40.

McBridge, C. M., Bowen, J. M. & Dmochowski, L. (1972) Antinuclear antibodies in the serum of patients with malignant melanoma. *Surgical Forum*, **23**, 92.

McCarthy, W. H. & Milton, G. W. (1975) Immunotherapy of malignant melanoma. *Behring Institute Mitteilungen*, **56**, 251.

McCulloch, P., Dent, P., Lui, V. *et al.* (1975) Improved survival in metastatic malignant melanoma with BCG therapy. *Proceedings of the American Association for Cancer Research*, **16**, 174.

McGovern, V. J. (1966) Melanoblastoma in Australia. In *Structure and Control of the Melanocyte*, p. 312. Berlin: Springer-Verlag.

McGovern, V. J. (1972) Melanoma; growth patterns, multiplicity and regression. In *Melanoma and Skin Cancer. Proceedings of the International Cancer Conference, Sydney, N.S.W.*, p. 95. Sydney: Government Printer.

McGovern, V. J. (1975) Spontaneous regression of melanoma. *Pathology*, **7**, 91.

McKenna, J. M., Sanderson, R. P. & Blakemore, W. S. (1964) Studies of antigens of human tumours. I. Demonstration of a soluble specific antigen in HeLa cells and some human tumours. *Cancer Research*, **24**, 754.

McLeod, G. R. (1972) Factors influencing prognosis in malignant melanoma. In *Melanoma and Skin Cancer. Proceedings of the International Cancer Conference, Sydney, N.S.W.*, p. 367. Sydney: Government Printer.

MacDonald, E. J. (1963) Epidemiology of melanoma. *Annals of the New York Academy of Sciences*, **100**, 4.

MacFadden, D. K., Lewis, M. G. & Rowden, G. (1976) Kidney deposition of immune complexes in malignancy. (Paper in preparation.)

Macher, E., Muller, C. H. R., Sorg, G., *et al.* (1975) Evidence for cross-reacting membrane-associated specific melanoma antigens as detected by immunofluorescence and immune adherence. *Behring Institute Mitteilungen*, **56**, 86.

Mackaness, G. A., Auclair, D. J. & Lagrange, P. (1973) Immunotherapy with BCG. I. Immune responses to different strains and preparations. *Journal of the National Cancer Institute*, **51**, 1655.

Mackie, R. M., Spilg, W. G. S., Thomas, C. E., *et al.* (1972) Cell-mediated immunity in patients with malignant melanoma. *British Journal of Dermatology*, **87**, 523.

MacLennon, I. C. M. & Harding, B. (1973) Some characteristics of immunoglobulins involved in antibody dependent lymphocyte cytotoxicity. *British Journal of Cancer*, **28**, 7.

Malek-Mansour, S., Castermans-Elias, S. & Lapiere, C. C. (1973) Regression de metastases de mélanome après thérapeutique immunologique. *Dermatologica*, **146**, 156.

Maluish, A. & Halliday, A. J. (1974) Cell-mediated immunity and specific serum factors in human cancer. The leucocyte adherence inhibition test. *Journal of the National Cancer Institute*, **52**, 1415.

Mann, D. L. (1975) An approach to the development of antisera to tumour associated antigens: experienc with acute leukemia and melanoma. *Behring Institute Mitteilungen*, **56**, 103.

Mansell, P. W. A., Krementz, E. T. & Diluzio, N. R. (1975) Clinical experience with immunotherapy of melanoma. *Behring Institute Mitteilungen*, **56**, 256.

Mastrangelo, M. J., Bellet, R. E., Berkelhammer, J., *et al.* (1975) Regression of pulmonary metastatic disease associated with intralesional BCG therapy of intracutaneous melanoma metastases. *Cancer*, **36**, 1305.

Mastrangelo, M. J., Berd, D. & Bellet, R. E. (1976) Critical review of previously reported clinical trials of cancer immunotherapy with non-specific immunostimulants. *Annals of the New York Academy of Sciences* (in press).

Mastrangelo, M. J., Laucius, J. F. & Outzen, H. C. (1975) Fundamental concepts in tumour immunology: a brief review. *Seminars in Oncology*, **1**, 291.

Mastrangelo, M. J., Sulit, H. L., Prehn, L. M., *et al.* (1975) Intralesional BCG in the treatment of metastatic malignant melanoma. *Cancer* (in press).

Mathè, G., Amiel, J. L., Schwartzenberg, L., *et al.* (1968) Demonstration of the efficacy of active immunotherapy in human acute lymphoblastic leukemia. *Revue européene d'études cliniques et biologiques*, **13**, 881.

Mavligit, G. M., Ambus, U., Gutterman, J. U., *et al.* (1973a) Antigens solubilized from human solid tumours: lymphocyte stimulation and cutaneous delayed sensitivity. *Nature (New Biology)*, **243**, 188.

Mavligit, G. M., Gutterman, J. U., McBride, C. M., *et al.* (1973b) Cell-mediated immunity to human solid tumours: *in vitro* detection by lymphocyte blastogenic responses to cell-associated and solubilized tumour antigens. *National Cancer Institute Monographs*, **37**, 167.

Metzgar, R. S., Bergoc, P. M., Moreno, M. A., *et al.* (1973) Melanoma antibodies produced by monkeys by immunization with human melanoma cell lines. *Journal of the National Cancer Institute*, **50**, 1065.

Milton, G. W. & Lane Brown, M. M. (1966) The limited role of attenuated smallpox virus in the management of advanced malignant melanoma. *Australian and New Zealand Journal of Surgery*, **35**, 268.

Milton, G. W., Lane Brown, M. M. & Gilder, M. (1967) Malignant melanoma with an occult primary lesion. *British Journal of Surgery*, **54**, 631.

Minton, J. R. (1973) Mumps virus and BCG vaccine in metastatic melanoma. *Archives of Surgery*, **106**, 503.

Mitchen, J. R., Moore, G. E., Gerner, R. E., *et al.* (1973) Interactions of human melanoma cell lines with autochthonous lymphoid cells. *Yale Journal of Biology and Medicine*, **46**, 669.

Moore, G. E. & Gerner, R. E. (1971) Malignant melanoma. *Surgery, Gynecology and Obstetrics*, **132**, 427.

Morton, D. L. (1971) Immunological studies with human neoplasms. *Journal of the Reticuloendothelial Society*, **10**, 137.

Morton, D. L. (1974) Cancer immunotherapy: an overview. *Seminars in Oncology*, **1**, 297.

Morton, D. L., Eilber, F. R., Malmgren, R. A., *et al.* (1970) Immunological factors which influence response to immunotherapy in malignant melanoma. *Surgery*, **68**, 158.

Morton, D. L., Eilber, F. R. & Malmgren, R. A. (1971) Immune factors in human cancer: malignant melanoma, skeletal and soft tissue sarcomas. *Progress in Experimental Tumour Research*, **14**, 25.

Morton, D. L., Eilber, F. R., Holmes, E. C., *et al.* (1974) BCG immunotherapy of malignant melanoma: summary of a seven year experience. *Annals of Surgery*, **180**, 635.

Morton, D. L., Malmgren, R. A., Holmes, E. C., *et al.* (1968) Demonstration of antibodies against human malignant melanoma by immunofluorescence. *Surgery*, **64**, 233.

Mukherji, B., Nathanson, L. & Clark, D. A. (1973) Studies of humoral and cell-mediated immunity in human melanoma. *Yale Journal of Biology and Medicine*, **46**, 681.

Muna, N. M., Marcus, S. & Smart, C. (1969) Detection by immunofluorescence of antibodies specific for human malignant melanoma cells. *Cancer*, **23**, 88.

Nadler, S. H. & Moore, G. E. (1965) Autotransplantation of human cancer. *Journal of the American Medical Association*, **191**, 105.

Nadler, S. H. & Moore, G. E. (1969) Immunotherapy of malignant disease. *Archives of Surgery*, **99**, 376.

Nagel, G. A. (1970) Immunité cellulaire du mélanome. *Revue de l'Institute Pasteur de Lyon*, **3**, 207.

Nairn, R. C. (1969) *Fluorescent Protein Tracing*, 3rd edition. Edinburgh: Churchill Livingstone.

Nairn, R. C. (1974) Malignant Melanoma. In *Immunological Aspects of Skin Diseases*, ed. Fry, L. & Seah, P. P., p. 153. Lancaster: Medical and Technical Publishing Co.

Nairn, R. C., Nind, A. P. P., Guli, E. P. G., *et al.* (1972) Anti-tumour immunoreactivity in patients with malignant melanoma. *Medical Journal of Australia*, **1**, 397.

Nathanson, L. (1972) Regression of intradermal melanoma after intralesional injection of *Mycobacterium bovis* strain of BCG. *Cancer Chemotherapy Report*, **56**, 659.

Nathanson, L. (1974) Use of BCG in the treatment of human neoplasms: a review. *Seminars in Oncology*, **1**, 337.

Nathanson, L., Necheles, T. F., Clark, D. A., *et al.* (1975) HL-A masking activity in malignant melanoma. *Behring Institute Mitteilungen*, **56**, 97.

Nind, A. P. P., Nairn, R. C., Rolland, J. M., *et al.* (1973) Lymphocyte anergy in patients with carcinoma. *British Journal of Cancer*, **28**, 108.

Oettgen, H. F., Aoki, T., Old, L. J., *et al.* (1968) Suspensions culture of a pigment-producing cell line derived from a human melanoma. *Journal of the National Cancer Institute*, **41**, 827.

Oettgen, H. F., Old, L. J. & Boyse, E. A. (1971) Human tumour immunology. *Medical Clinics of North America*, **55**, 761.

Old, L. J. & Boyse, E. A. (1965) Antigens of tumours and leukaemias induced by viruses. *Federation Proceedings*, **24**, 1009.

Old, L. J., Clarke, D. A. & Benacerrof, B. (1959) Effects of Bacillus Calmette-Guérin infection on transplanted tumours in the mouse. *Nature* (Suppl. 5), **184**, 291.

O'Neill, P. A. & Romsdahl, M. M. (1974) IgA as a blocking factor in human malignant melanoma. *Immunological Communications*, **3**, 427.

Oon, C. J., Apsey, M., Buckleton, H., *et al.* (1975) Human immune γ-globulin treated with chlorambucil for cancer therapy. *Behring Institute Mitteilungen*, **56**, 228.

Oon, C. J., Butterworth, C. Elliott, P., *et al.* (1975) Homologous immunotherapy using immune leukocytes. *Behring Institute Mitteilungen*, **56**, 223.

O'Toole, C., Perlmann, P., Unsgaard, B., *et al.* (1972) Cellular immunity to human urinary bladder carcinoma: correlation to clinical stage and radiotherapy. *International Journal of Cancer*, **10**, 77.

O'Toole, C., Stejskal, V., Perlmann, P., *et al.* (1974) Lymphoid cell mediating tumour-specific cytotoxicity to carcinoma of the urinary bladder. *Journal of Experimental Medicine*, **139**, 457.

Pack, G. T. (1950) Quoted by Nagel, G., Piessons, W. F. Stilmant, M. M., *et al.* (1971) Evidence for tumour-specific immunity in human malignant melanoma. *European Journal of Cancer*, **7**, 41.

Pack, G. T. & Miller, T. R. (1961) Metastatic melanoma with indeterminate primary site. *Journal of the American Medical Association*, **176**, 55.

Parsons, P. G., Goss, P. & Pope, J. H. (1974) Detection in human melanoma cell lines of particles with some properties common with RNA-tumour viruses. *International Journal of Cancer*, **13**, 606.

Pavie-Fischer, J., Kourilsky, F. M., Banzet, P., *et al.* (1975) Investigation of cell-mediated immune reactions in malignant melanoma using the chromium release test. *Behring Institute Mitteilungen*, **56**, 160.

Peter, H. H., Diehl, V., Kalden, J. R., *et al.* (1975) Humoral and cellular cytotoxicity *in vitro* against allogeneic and autologous human melanoma cells. *Behring Institute Mitteilungen*, **56**, 167.

Petersen, N. C., Bodenham, D. C. & Lloyd, O. C. (1962) Malignant melanomas of the skin. *British Journal of Plastic Surgery*, **15**, 49.

Phillips, T. M. (1971) Immunofluorescent techniques in the study of malignant melanoma. *Revue de l'Institute Pasteur de Lyon*, **4**, 331.

Phillips, T. M. & Lewis, M. G. (1970) A system of immunofluorescence in the study of tumour cells. *Revue européene d'études cliniques et biologiques*, **15**, 1016.

Pihl, E., Nind, A. P. P. & Nairn, R. C. (1974) Electron microscope observation of the *in vitro* interactions between human leucocytes and cancer cells. *Australian Journal of Experimental Biology and Medical Science*, **52**, 737

Pilch, Y. H., Fritze, D. & Kern, D. H. (1975) Immune cytolysis of human melanoma cells mediated by immune RNA. *Behring Institute Mitteilungen*, **56**, 184.

Pilch, Y. H., Veltman, L. L. & Kern, D. H. (1974) Immune cytolysis of human tumour cells mediated by xenogeneic 'immune' RNA: implications for immunotherapy. *Surgery*, **76**, 23.

Pinsky, C. M., Hirshaut, Y. & Oettgen, H. F. (1973) Treatment of malignant melanoma by intralesional injection of BCG. *National Cancer Institute Monographs*, **39**, 225.

Ploem, J. S. (1970) Quantitative immunofluorescence. In *Standardization in Immunofluorescence*, ed. Holborow, E. J. Ch. 10, p. 63. Oxford: Blackwell.

Poskitt, P. K. F., Poskitt, T. R. & Wallace, J. H. (1974) Renal deposition of soluble immune complexes in mice bearing B-16 melanoma. *Journal of Experimental Medicine*, **140**, 410.

Prehn, R. T. (1972) The immune reaction as a stimulator of tumour growth. *Science* (N.Y.), **176**, 170.

Prehn, R. T. & Main, J. M. (1957) Immunity to methylcholanthrene-induced sarcomas. *Journal of the National Cancer Institute*, **18**, 769.

Proctor, J. W., Thomson, D. M. P., Stokowski, L., *et al.* (1976) Immunoglobulins are not detected on the surface of tumour cells within rat sarcomas. (Paper in preparation.)

Pulvertaft, R. T. V. (1959) The examination of pathological tissue in a fresh state. In *Modern Trends in Pathology*, ed. Collins, D. H., p. 19. London, Butterworth.

Rahi, A. H. S. (1971) Autoimmune reactions in uveal melanoma. *British Journal of Ophthalmology*, **55**, 792.

Riethmüller, G., Saal, J. G., Ehinger, H., *et al.* (1975) Cell-mediated cytotoxicity in patients with malignant melanoma treated with BCG. *Behring Institute Mitteilungen*, **56**, 177.

Ritchers, A. & Kaspersky, C. L. (1975) Surface immunoglobulin-positive lymphocytes in human breast cancer tissue and homolateral axillary lymph nodes. *Cancer*, **35**, 129.

Roberts, M. M., Bass, E. M., Wallace, I. W., *et al.* (1973) Local immunoglobulin production in breast cancer. *British Journal of Cancer*, **27**, 269.

Roenigk, H. H., Deodhar, S. D., Krebs, J. A., *et al.* (1975) Microcytotoxicity and serum blocking factors in malignant melanoma and halo naevus. *Archives of Dermatology*, **111**, 720.

Romsdahl, M. M. & Cox, I. S. (1970) Human malignant melanoma antibodies demonstrated by immunofluorescence. *Archives of Surgery*, **100**, 491.

Romsdahl, M. M. & Cox, I. S. (1971) Evidence for enhancing antibodies in human sarcomas. *Proceedings of the American Association for Cancer Research*, **12**, 66.

Roubin, R., Césarini, J. P., Fridman, W. H., *et al.* (1975) Characterization of the mononuclear cell infiltrate in human malignant melanoma. *International Journal of Cancer*, **16**, 61.

Rowden, G. & Lewis, M. G. (1975a) Immunological and ultra-structural investigations of halo naevi. *Proceedings of the Microscopical Society of Canada*, **2**, 24.

Rowden, G. & Lewis, M. G. (1975b) Foetal-associated and tumour-specific antigens of cultured malignant melanoma cells: An electron microscope immunocytochemical study. *Proceedings of the 9th International Pigment Cell Biological Conference* (Houston). Berlin: Karger (in press).

Roy, C., Lewis, M. G., Capek, A., *et al.* (1976) Studies of cytotoxic lymphocytes in patients with malignant melanoma. (Paper in preparation.)

Saval, H. (1969) Effects of autologous extracts on cultivated human peripheral blood lymphocytes. *Cancer*, **24**, 56.

Segall, A., Weiler, O., Genin, J., *et al.* (1972) *In vitro* study of cellular immunity against human cancer. *International Journal of Cancer*, **9**, 417.

Seigler, H. F., Shingleton, W. W., Horne, B. J., *et al.* (1975) The use of BCG, adoptive transfer and neuraminidase-treated tumour cells in the management of melanoma. *Behring Institute Mitteilungen*, **56**, 214.

Seigler, H. F., Shingleton, W. W., Metzgar, R. S., *et al.* (1972) Nonspecific and specific immunotherapy in patients with melanoma. *Surgery*, **72**, 162.

Seigler, H. F., Shingleton, W. W., Metzgar, R. S., *et al.* (1973) Immunotherapy in patients with melanoma. *Annals of Surgery*, **178**, 352.

Seigler, H. F., Shingleton, W. W. & Pickrell, K. L. (1975) Intralesional BCG, intravenous immune lymphocytes and immunization with neuraminidase-treated tumour cells to manage melanoma: a clinical assessment. *Plastic and Reconstructive Surgery*, **55**, 294.

Serrow, B., Michel, H., Dubois, J. B., *et al.* (1975) Granulomatous hepatitis caused by BCG infection during immunotherapy of a malignant melanoma. *Biomedicine*, **23**, 236.

Shibata, H., Jerry, L. M., Lewis, M. G., *et al.* (1976) Specific anti-tumour immune reactions in patients following autoimmunisation and oral BCG. *Cancer* (in press).

Simmons, R. L. (1972) Quoted by Morton, D. L., Haskell, C. M., Pilch, Y. H., *et al*. Recent advances in Oncology: UCLA Conference. *Annals of Internal Medicine*, 77, 431.

Simmons, R. L. & Rios, A. (1971) Combined use of BCG and neuraminidase in experimental tumour immunotherapy. *Surgical Forum*, 22, 99.

Sjögren, H. O., Hellström, I., Bansal, S. C., *et al*. (1971) Suggestive evidence that blocking antibodies of tumour bearing individuals may be antigen–antibody complexes. *Proceedings of the National Academy of Sciences* (Washington), 68, 1372.

Sjörgren, H. O., Hellström, I., Bansal, S. C., *et al*. (1972) Elution of 'blocking factors' from human tumours, capable of abrogating tumour cell destruction by specifically immune lymphocytes. *International Journal of Cancer*, 9, 274.

Smith, G. V., Morse, P. A., Deraps, G. D., *et al*. (1973) Immunotherapy of patients with cancer. *Surgery*, 74, 59.

Smith, J. L. & Stehlin, J. S. (1965) Spontaneous regression of primary malignant melanoma with regional metastases. *Cancer*, 18, 1399.

Smithers, D. (1971) Some tumour behaviour patterns which may illuminate the cancer process. *British Cancer Council, 3rd Symposium, Cancer Priorities*, p. 30. London: George and Chase.

Sparks, F. C., Silverstein, M. J., Hunt, J. S., *et al*. (1973) Complications of BCG immunotherapy in patients with cancer. *New England Journal of Medicine*, 289, 827.

Spitler, L. E., Wybran, J., Fudenberg, H. H., *et al*. (1972) Transfer factor therapy of malignant melanoma. Abstracts of the *Journal of Clinical Investigation*, 51, 92a.

Spitler, L. E., Wybran, J., Fudenberg, H. H., *et al*. (1973) Transfer factor therapy in malignant melanoma. *Clinical Research*, 21, 221.

Stegmaier, O. C., Becker, S. W., Jr & Medenica, M. (1969) Multiple halo naevi. *Archives of Dermatology*, 99, 180.

Stephens, O. E. A. (1966) Quoted by Boyd, W. in *The Spontaneous Regression of Cancer*. Philadelphia: Saunders.

Stewart, T. H. M. (1969) The presence of delayed hypersensitivity reactions in patients towards cellular extracts of their malignant tumours. *Cancer*, 23, 1368.

Stjernswärd, J., Clifford, B., Singh, S., *et al*. (1968) Indication of cellular immunological reactions against autochthonous tumours in cancer patients studied *in vitro*. *East African Medical Journal*, 45, 484.

Stjernswärd, J. & Levin, A. (1971) Delayed hypersensitivity induced regression of human neoplasms. *Cancer*, 28, 628.

Stuhlmiller, G. M. & Seigler, H. F. (1975) Characterization of a chimpanzee anti-human melanoma antiserum. *Cancer Research*, 35, 2132.

Sumner, W. C. & Foraker, A. G. (1960) Spontaneous regression of human melanoma: clinical and experimental studies. *Cancer*, 13, 79.

Sutton, R. L. (1916) An unusual variety of vitiligo: leukoderma acquisitum centrifugum. *Journal of Cutaneous Diseases*, 34, 797.

Takasugi, M. & Klein, E. (1970) A microassay for cell-mediated immunity. *Transplantation*, 9, 219.

Takasugi, M., Mickey, M. R. & Takasugi, I. (1973) Reactivity of lymphocytes from normal persons on tissue culture tumour cells. *Cancer Research*, 33, 2898.

Takasugi, M., Mickey, M. R. & Teraski, P. I. (1974) Studies of the specificity of cell-mediated immunity to human tumours. *Journal of the National Cancer Institute*, 53, 1527.

Teimourian, B. & McCune, W. S. (1963) Surgical management of malignant melanoma. *American Journal of Surgery*, 29, 529.

The, T. H., Eibergen, R., Lamberts, H. B., *et al*. (1972) Immune phagocytosis *in vivo* of human malignant melanoma cells. *Acta medica scandinavica*, 192, 141.

The, T. H., Huiges, H. A., Schraffordt-Koops, H., *et al*. (1975) Surface antigens on cultured malignant melanoma cells as detected by a membrane immunofluorescence method with human sera. Lack of tumour-specific reactions on melanoma lines. *Annals of the New York Academy of Sciences*, 254, 528.

Thompson, P. G. (1972) The relationship of lymphocytic infiltration to progress in primary malignant melanoma of the skin. *Eighth International Pigment Cell Biology Conference, I.U.A.C., Sydney, Australia*, p. 100. Sydney: Government Printer.

Tisman, G., Wu, S. J. G. & Safire, G. E. (1975) Intralesional PPD in malignant melanoma. *Lancet*, i, 161.

Todd, D. W., Spencer-Payne, W., Farrow, G. M., *et al*. (1966) Spontaneous regression of primary malignant melanoma with regional metastases: report of a case with photographic documentation. *Proceedings of the Mayo Clinic*, 41, 10.

Underwood, J. C. E. (1974) Lymphoreticular infiltration in human tumours: prognostic and biological implications. A review. *British Journal of Cancer*, 30, 538.

Underwood, J. C. E. & Carr, I. (1972) The ultrastructure of the lymphoreticular cells in non-lymphoid neoplasms. *Virchows Archiv für Pathologisch Anatomie und für klinische Medizin*, 12, 39.

Van Den Brenk, H. A. S. (1969) Autoimmunization in human malignant melanoma. *British Medical Journal*, iv, 171.

Vennegoor, D. & Van Smeerdijk, D. (1975) Effects of mixtures and complexes of chlorambucil and antibody on a human melanoma cell line. *European Journal of Cancer*, 11, 725.

Veronesi, U., Cascinelli, N., Fossati, G., *et al*. (1973) Lymphocyte toxicity test in clinical melanoma. *European Journal of Cancer*, 9, 843.

Virchow, R. (1863) *Krankhaften Geschwulste.* Cited by Underwood (1974).

Viza, D. & Phillips, J. (1971) Extraction and solubilization of cell surface antigens from malignant melanoma. *Revue de l'Institute Pasteur de Lyon*, **4,** 339.

Viza, D., Phillips, J. & Trejdosiewicz, L. K. (1975) Cell surface and serum associated antigens. *Behring Institute Mitteilungen*, **56,** 83.

Voisin, G. A., Kinsky, R. G. & Jansen, F. K. (1966) Transplantation immunity: localization in mouse serum of antibodies responsible for haemagglutination, cytotoxicity and enhancement. *Nature (Lond.),* **210,** 138.

Wade, H. (1908) An experimental investigation of infective sarcoma in the dog, with a consideration of its relationship to cancer. *Journal of Pathology and Bacteriology*, **12,** 384.

Warren, B. A. (1973) Environment of the blood borne tumour embolus adherent to vessel wall. *Journal of Medicine*, **4,** 150.

Wayte, D. M. & Helwig, E. G. (1968) Halo naevi. *Cancer, N.Y.*, **22,** 69.

Whitehouse, J. M. A. (1973) Circulating antibodies in human malignant disease. *British Journal of Cancer*, **28,** 170.

Whitehouse, J. M. A. & Holborow, E. S. (1971) Smooth muscle antibody in malignant disease. *British Medical Journal*, iv, 511.

Wilbur, D. L. & Hartmann, H. P. (1931) Malignant melanoma with delayed metastatic growth. *Annals of Internal Medicine*, **5,** 201.

Williams, J. W., Davies, K., Jones, W. M., *et al.* (1968) Malignant melanoma of the skin: Prognostic value of histology. *British Journal of Cancer*, **22,** 452.

Witz, I. P. (1973) The biological significance of tumour-bound immunoglobulins. *Current Topics in Microbiology and Immunology*, **61,** 151.

Woglom, W. H. (1929) Immunity to transplantable tumours. *Cancer Reviews*, **4,** 129.

Wood, G. W. & Barth, R. F. (1974) Immunofluorescent studies of the serological reactivity of patients with malignant melanoma against tumour-associated cytoplasmic antigens. *Journal of the National Cancer Institute*, **53,** 309.

Wood, S., Jr (1958) Pathogenesis of metastasis formation observed *in vivo* in the rabbit ear chamber. *Archives of Pathology (and Laboratory Medicine)*, **66,** 550.

Wood, S., Jr (1964) Experimental studies of the intravascular dissemination of ascites V2 carcinoma cells in the rabbit with special reference to fibrinogen and fibrinolytic agents. *Bulletin der Schweizerischen Akademie der Medizinischen Wissenschaften* (Basel), **20,** 92.

Wood, S., Jr (1973) *The Microcirculation in Clinical Medicine*, ed. Wells, R., p. 275. New York: Academic Press.

11. Melanoma in Pregnancy; Occult Primary Melanoma; Melanoma in Children; Spontaneous Regression

MELANOMA IN PREGNANCY

The relationship between melanoma and pregnancy can best be considered under three major headings.

1. THE SYMPTOMS (p. 56)

The symptoms caused by the majority of malignant melanomas arising in pregnancy are the same as those caused by the disease at other times. However, there are two exceptions to this rule which occur so rarely that it is difficult to decide whether they are coincidental or related to the pregnancy. First, a prominent feature of several primary melanomas in pregnant women has been a marked itch in the vicinity of the lesion which seems more pronounced than the irritation observed in other patients; consequently, I (G. W. M.) think it is wise to biopsy (p. 34) any 'mole' causing irritation in pregnancy. Second, I have seen four cases in whom a lesion has enlarged during pregnancy and regressed after delivery of the baby. The most definite case of this was a young woman who, during three pregnancies, developed an enlarging amelanotic nodule on her cheek, and after each delivery the lesion regressed. Immediately after the third pregnancy, the lesion was biopsied and reported as amelanotic malignant melanoma; it was then excised with a margin and the patient has remained well and free of disease for three years.

Most junctional naevi tend to darken and enlarge during pregnancy, but this change affects *all* lesions and should not cause alarm; it is the growth of a single lesion which demands a diagnosis.

2. CLINICAL SIGNS

The clinical signs of melanoma in pregnancy are in no way exceptional to those of melanoma in general.

3. PROGNOSIS

The effect of pregnancy on the prognosis of malignant melanoma can be subdivided into:

a. The effect of pregnancy on a small primary lesion.

b. The effect of pregnancy in precipitating recurrence after apparently effective treatment.

a. There have only been 12 cases of pregnant women developing primary malignant melanoma in this series, and the pattern of behaviour of the disease, as a rule, is in no way exceptional. It appears as if the melanoma is often detected at an early stage because the young woman is attending her obstetrician at regular intervals. An exception to this are the four cases referred to above, where the primary lesion regressed after delivery; in these cases the behaviour of the melanoma appeared to be intimately affected by the pregnancy.

b. The prognosis of an apparently cured melanoma could be worsened if pregnancy caused a sudden recrudescence of the disease. My figures are inadequate to prove this, because although there are occasional women who soon after becoming pregnant have a flare-up of their malignant melanoma, the number is no higher than similar but apparently spontaneous flare-ups of tumour which occur in men. Indeed one man in this series survived in perfect health for 24 years before developing widespread and rapidly fatal melanoma.

Questions are often asked in relation to the management of melanoma in pregnancy.

Q. *Should a pregnancy be terminated?*

A. It is not definitely known whether melanoma in pregnancy carries a slightly worse prognosis than melanoma at other times of life. If a primary melanoma is discovered after the fetus is viable, then an induction of labour followed in a few weeks by definitive treatment of the melanoma appears to be a reasonable course of action. If the small primary lesion is diagnosed in the early months of pregnancy, wide excision and either graft or primary wound closure is carried out; at each visit to her obstetrician, the site of the melanoma excision, intransit areas and the draining lymph nodes are examined. The treatment of these, if they should become enlarged, would depend on the circumstances at the time.

Note: The average time between the removal of the primary and clinically involved lymph nodes is 19·9 months. Hence, the woman should be able to complete her pregnancy without clinical involvement of lymph nodes. The pregnancy should be terminated under one circumstance—if the melanoma has become widely disseminated and it is unlikely that the mother will survive until the baby is viable.

Q. *Should a young woman allow herself to become pregnant after the apparently successful removal of a primary melanoma?*

A. Although I believe that pregnancy is unlikely to precipitate a recurrence of the melanoma, this is not yet proven. Therefore, in young women it would probably be sensible to wait three years before pregnancy because the majority of locally recurring disease does so in that time. Older women who feel that their opportunities for child bearing are diminishing can be advised that the case against pregnancy is not proved; there may be a slight risk but if the mother is prepared to accept it, the chance of a flare-up of her melanoma is not great.

Q. A question sometimes asked by a young pregnant woman: '*If I have this baby, is there any chance that the baby may have the growth too?*'

A. It has been reported that melanoma can spread from the mother to the fetus. However, it is by no means certain that this will occur and in those patients I have seen (three) with extensive tumour, the child in each case did not have evidence of disease.

OCCULT PRIMARY MELANOMA

The presentation of occult primary melanoma is discussed on page 29. The overall incidence of occult primary melanoma is difficult to assess in a special unit. The incidence reported in the literature varies from 1 to 8 per cent and is probably less than 5 per cent (Pack and Miller, 1961; Das Gupta, Bowden and Berg, 1963; Mundth, Guralnick and Raker, 1965; Smith and Stehlin, 1965; Beardmore, 1972). In all figures, the incidence in men is higher than in women. In our figures, the ratio is about 4·6 : 1 (32 men and 7 women); while in those reported by Beardmore, the ratio is 2 : 1. The average age of the patients with occult primary melanoma is 45·4 years, i.e. the same as the average age of presentation of melanoma. The youngest patient was 18 and the oldest 78 at the time of diagnosis.

The 39 patients in this series can be divided into two groups. Eighteen patients (13 men, 5 women) were true occult primary patients because there was no history of any lesion which could have been a primary melanoma and none was discovered during treatment. In 21 patients (19 men, 2 women) a history was obtained of a lesion which could have been a primary melanoma, e.g. the patient had noticed a 'blood blister' in an area draining into the enlarged nodes, the blister was either slightly injured or became 'infected', i.e. red and inflamed, and then fell off or just 'disappeared'. Table 11.1 shows the site of the lymph node involvement.

In nine men, the metastasis was not in a major lymph node group (indeterminate group). One man had generalised disease from the first diagnosis, i.e. multiple subcutaneous

Table 11.1 The site of enlarged lymph nodes in patients with occult primary melanoma. Indeterminate indicates that the first detected tumour was either central (blood borne) or involved multiple lymph node sites from the outset

	Neck	Axilla	Groin	Indeterminate
Men	7	8	8	9
Women	2	2	3	—

nodules, and the remaining eight had subcutaneous nodules which could have been either intransit metastases or subcutaneous blood borne metastases.

The survival of patients who have an occult primary melanoma is certainly not good. Of the 32 men, 17 are known to have died of melanoma between 6 and 84 months after the lesion was diagnosed. Two patients were last seen 12 and 13 months after diagnosis was established; both had extensive metastases but we have no record of their death. Nine patients are alive and free of all sign of melanoma for an average time of 45 months, the range being 19 to 81 months. Two patients are alive but known to have metastatic tumour 6 and 31 months after the diagnosis. One patient has been lost to follow-up. From these figures it would appear that a man who presents with an occult primary melanoma and metastasis has roughly one chance in three of surviving.

The number of women with occult primary melanoma is less, and the figures therefore have less significance. Two women have died, one 23 months and the other 26 months after diagnosis. However, one of these women died of a coronary occlusion and had no evidence of disease when she died. Four women are alive, well and free of evidence of disease; the average survival is 76 months, the range being 49 to 91 months. One woman is alive eight months after diagnosis but has evidence of recurrent melanoma. It is evident from these figures that the survival of women with occult primary melanoma is likely to be better than the survival of men. This agrees with the usual survival figures of melanoma.

TREATMENT

The following factors are relevant to the selection of treatment:

1. If no evidence of the primary lesion is discovered at the time of the initial treatment, then it will almost certainly never be detected.

2. Many of these patients are in the prime of life.

3. The prognosis, although bad, is not hopeless.

4. For practical purposes, those patients with lymph node metastasis may be considered as having a cured primary lesion who develop nodal deposits. Hence, other factors being equal, a radical lymph node resection involving the site of the palpable nodes is carried out. This is supported by the fact that in 16 patients who had lymph node biopsy examination of the specimen involved after radical resection revealed one or more remaining nodes also involved with the tumour.

5. The nine patients who had occult primary melanoma with systemic and not nodal metastasis all died within less than 12 months of diagnosis of the disease.

MELANOMA IN CHILDREN

Melanoma in children is, fortunately, a rare condition. I have been responsible at one stage or another for the care of six children under 10 years of age. This is not an adequate number to produce useful statistics. However, the six cases seen at the Melanoma Unit of Sydney Hospital illustrate some of the difficulties which may be seen with this disease in children.

1. There is a very natural reluctance to carry out surgery, which a child may feel is horribly mutilating.

2. The great rarity of the condition implies that even if the clinician thinks of the diagnosis, the pathologist, once he sees the age of the patient, may be reluctant to commit himself to malignant melanoma as a diagnosis.

3. The symptomatology of melanoma in children is similar to that in the adult age group. A proportion of the lesions show no pigment while most seem to be darkly

coloured. The usual symptoms of enlargement, itch and bleeding are prominent in childhood, while the duration of symptoms, i.e. measured in months from the change of a pre-existing lesion, is also similar to that which occurs in the older age group.

4. The progress of the disease in children is usually described as having a course similar to that in adults, but the course in these children is remarkable, one child evidently having had a temporary spontaneous regression.

5. Even the experienced pathologist may have great difficulty in early cases determining whether in fact the lesion is a malignant melanoma.

6. Palpation of normal lymph nodes in people can cause great difficulty in detecting early spread of the disease. This applies particularly in adolescents in whom acne can cause slight enlargement of the draining nodes, so that an early detection of metastasis can be nearly impossible. There have been two teenagers not reported in this chapter, in whom definite enlargement was, in retrospect, due to mild acne in the draining area, although when the nodes first became palpable, they were thought to be possibly metastatic melanoma because they were not tender. Careful palpation of the inguinal region in children will usually detect two or three flat, bean-shaped nodes.

The plan of action which has been evolved with these children is as follows:

1. Establish the diagnosis by excision biopsy and paraffin sections. The sections are shown to three pathologists independently and the age is withheld until the pathologist is satisfied with the diagnosis. If, in spite of this, the opinion of the pathologists is not unanimous and there is continuing doubt about the diagnosis, the treatment consists of wide local excision, no skin graft, i.e. primary closure *and* careful follow-up for five years.

2. If the diagnosis is unequivocally established and the lesion shows the unfavourable characteristic of deep penetration into the dermis, then, provided there is no sign of general dissemination, a prophylactic lymph node dissection has been carried out, if possible, in continuity with the site of the primary lesion. It is important that both the child and the parents fully understand the reasons for the proposed course of therapy. Of the six cases I have seen, three have died and three remain alive three years after treatment.

SPONTANEOUS REGRESSION (Medical Journal of Australia, 1975)

'Spontaneous' (Shorter Oxford English Dictionary): '1. arising, proceeding or acting entirely from natural impulse, without any external stimulus or constraint; voluntary. 2. of natural processes; having a self-contained cause or origin'.

Spontaneous regression of a malignant process is always a matter of interest to students of disease. Spontaneous regression of cancer is also tantalising because the cause of the regression remains elusive. Everson and Cole (1966), in their classic study of the world experience, were unable to explain the phenomenon. I cannot offer any more reasonable speculations than those already advanced.

Spontaneous regression of malignant melanoma may take one of two forms. Regression of part or all of the primary tumour is quite common, i.e. about one patient in 20 will have no detectable primary tumour and at least three times this number will have demonstrable regression of part of the primary tumour (McGovern, 1975) (p. 17). Permanent regression of well-established metastases is far less common. One case in this series, a man known to have multiple small bowel secondaries, has lived in good health apparently free of disease for more than five years. Several other patients have had temporary regression or retrogression of demonstrable metastasis for up to 18 months, but the disease finally overcame them and was fatal.

The cause of the regression in both types is probably related to the host/tumour immunological balance, but when regression occurs there do not appear to be any obvious trigger mechanisms present either in the host or in the tumour. Some trigger mechanisms must exist in spite of the fact that we do not yet know how to recognise them.

COMMENT

The commonest form of spontaneous regression of a malignant melanoma occurs while the primary tumour is small; hence presumably it occurs because some part of the evolving tumour becomes antigenic to the host and is destroyed by immune mechanisms. The second and much rarer form of spontaneous regression occurs with advanced disease, although small metastases might be—indeed probably are—frequently destroyed by the host, but there is no way to detect this event. Everson and Cole (1966) reviewed and reported cases of this form of regression and suggested that the incidence of spontaneous regression was less than 0·5 per cent. In the series reported here, the incidence is about 0·1 per cent or less.

If a patient has a spontaneous regression of melanoma of established metastasis, two events must have occurred. Firstly, the original tumour must have formed, grown to a diagnosable size and then spread and grown again. At all stages of this process any tumour cell triggering the host resistance would be destroyed, so a population of non-antigenic tumour cells becomes established. Secondly, for some reason the tumour is either destroyed by the host or dies of causes within itself. If the tumour is destroyed by the host, then presumably the tumour becomes antigenic and indeed some of the reported cases have been associated with infection. However, this is not invariable and the common event in spontaneous regression is the tumour simply melts away without any simultaneous violent reaction in the host.

Another explanation of spontaneous regression is mis-diagnosis. The cases reported by Everson and Cole (1966) all had most convincing evidence for the diagnosis of advanced tumour, and in my cases, the diagnosis also appeared to be beyond doubt.

The answer to the riddle of spontaneous regression, like the answer to many other cancer problems, need not be the same factor in every case. In some patients the cause of the regression may lie in the tumour; in others it could be the host.

REFERENCES

Beardmore, G. L. (1972) The epidemiology of malignant melanoma in Australia. In *Melanoma and Skin Cancer. Proceedings of the International Cancer Conference*, ed. McCarthy, W. H., p. 39. Sydney: Government Printer.
Das Gupta, T., Bowden, L. & Berg, J. W. (1963) Malignant melanoma of unknown primary origin. *Surgery, Gynecology and Obstetrics*, **117**, 341.
Everson, T. C. & Cole, W. H. (1966) *Spontaneous Regression of Cancer; a Study and Abstract of Reports in the World Medical Literature and of Personal Communications concerning spontaneous regression of malignant disease*. Ch. 4. Philadelphia: Saunders.
McGovern, V. J. (1975) Spontaneous regression of melanoma. *Pathology*, 7, 91.
Medical Journal of Australia (1975) Editorial. *Medical Journal of Australia*, **2**, 761.
Mundth, E. D., Guralnick, E. A. & Raker, J. W. (1965) Malignant melanoma; a clinical study of 427 cases. *Annals of Surgery*, **162**, 15.
Pack, G. T. & Miller, T. R. (1961) Metastatic melanoma with inter-determinate primary site. Report of two instances of long term survival. *Journal of the American Medical Association*, **176**, 55.
Smith, J. L. & Stehlin, J. S. (1965) Spontaneous regression of primary malignant melanomas with regional metastases. *Cancer*, **18**, 1399.

12. Melanoma of the Nose and Mouth

Primary malignant melanoma in the mucosa of the nose and mouth is a rare disease, i.e. the incidence is between 1 and 2 per cent of all patients with melanoma (Milton and Lane Brown, 1965; Stewart, Hay and Varco, 1953; Charalambidis and Patterson, 1962; Daland, 1959; Moore and Martin, 1955; Pack, Gerber and Scharnagel, 1952; Kragh and Erich, 1960; Conley and Pack, 1963). It is a disease which usually carries a poor prognosis. It is also a disease which, in the mouth at any rate, could occasionally have a better outlook if the danger of a black or brown pigmented patch on the mucosa was appreciated.

Primary melanoma of the oro-nasal mucosa is so rare that statistical evaluation becomes difficult because of the small number of cases. Chaudhry, Hampel and Gorlin (1958) traced 105 published cases, the male to female incidence being 2 : 1. The commonest site was the palate with 80 per cent of the lesions, and after this in order of frequency came the lower jaw, cheek and tongue. Kragh and Erich (1960) reported four lesions on the upper jaw or hard palate and two on the tongue. However, Chaudhry et al. (1958) pointed out that it may be difficult to determine the exact site of origin with extensive lesions.

The present chapter deals only with mucosal melanoma of the nose and mouth. Lesions occurring on the skin and at the mucocutaneous junction (Smuts, 1939) are excluded. In 300 malignant tumours in the nose Stewart (1951) had an incidence of malignant melanoma of 4 per cent. This incidence is somewhat higher than that of Capps and Williams (1950) of one in 77 nasal cancers. Grace (1947) found 66 cases in the literature up to 1947 and reported the first case in a Negro. By 1960 Ravid and Esteves were able to trace 117 cases of intranasal malignant melanoma. The great majority of these cases originated in either the lower part of the septum or the middle and inferior turbinates; as in patients reported by Morey (1952), only four cases originated in the paranasal sinuses.

Hart reported a case (1943) in which a malignant melanoma arising in the skin of the back metastasised 10 years later in the sphenoidal sinus. The origin of malignant melanoma from the lower part of the nose is a little surprising because, as has been pointed out (Willis, 1948; Allen and Spitz, 1953; Ravid and Esteves, 1960), pigmentation in this region is very unusual, it being much more frequent to find pigmentation in the olfactory area.

The racial incidence of malignant melanoma in the mouth relative to malignant melanoma at other sites is of some interest. As Schoolman and Anderson (1950) have shown some pigmentation in the mouth is common in dark-skinned people. Prinz (1932) states that the oral pigmentation in Negroes is usually about the gums, in Eastern Europeans and gypsies pigmentation usually occurs in the gums and cheek. In any race the commonest site for oral malignant melanoma, i.e. the palate, is not markedly pigmented. Chaudhry et al. (1958) comment that it is difficult to determine the racial incidence, but in 73 of their oral cases, the race of the patient had been recorded and two of these were Negroes. None of Hewer's (1935) 47 cases of malignant melanoma among the Sudanese had an oral primary lesion. Baxter (1939) found 170 cases of malignant melanoma reported in dark-skinned races in whom the site of origin was specified, and Morris and Horn (1951) had 287 cases, and the primary lesion was in the mouth in eight (2·8 per cent). Lesions in the leg accounted for between 60 and 70 per cent of cases. The incidence of oral melanoma relative to cutaneous lesions in dark-skinned races may be slightly higher than in Caucasians.

Pigmentation in the mouth of many dogs is much more marked than in humans. The incidence of oral malignant melanoma appears to be higher in dog than in man. Cotchin (1955) reported 101 cases of melanotic tumours in dogs and 15 per cent of these were in the mouth. In 19 lesions reported by Mulligan (1949), six were in the palate or cheek. The incidence in the buccal mucosa relative to the palate is higher in dogs than in man (Povar and Povar, 1950). These observations suggest that inherited oral pigmentation in man does not greatly increase the risk of malignant melanoma. However, in dogs melanosis of the mouth definitely predisposes to malignant change.

Trauma

The role of trauma as an initiating cause of oral malignant melanoma has been the subject of much speculation. Several cases have been reported which appeared to be caused by different types of injury, e.g. a blow which dislodged a tooth (Greene *et al.*, 1954), cauterisation of patches of oral pigment (Sirsat, 1953), and suspected injury from cleaning the teeth (Friedrich and Renaud, 1960; Villa and Laico, 1961). However, in spite of these examples, I believe that trauma is unlikely to initiate malignant degeneration, although it may draw attention to an already malignant lesion. My reasons are:

1. No case has been reported where chronic irritation from a malfitting denture was the site of malignant change.

2. The lesions are as frequently situated on the centre of the palate as they are close to the teeth, thus the effect of cleaning the teeth is not marked.

3. Sirsat (1953), reporting a case of oral melanoma from Bombay, had three lesions in the roof of the mouth. These cases came from a country where betel nut chewing is a frequent habit and buccal carcinoma is common. Pigmentation of the buccal mucosa is also common. If trauma was an important cause of oral melanoma, then the incidence of the buccal mucosa should be high where a known irritant is at work; this is not so.

Clinical features

MOUTH

The clinical course of malignant melanoma in the mouth appears to develop in two stages. Initially, there is usually a period of flat, slowly enlarging, symptomless pigmentation, usually on the palate or upper alveolus (i.e. horizontal growth). In two of my cases, oral pigmentation had been known to be present for eight years.

At some stage the pattern of growth changes; the flat pigmented patches become rough, raised, nodular, friable and haemorrhagic. The speed of this vertical enlargement seems to vary considerably; the growth may be detectable over a few weeks, months or even up to five years. Once the growth pattern has changed, the friability and bleeding are usually marked (New and Hansel, 1921; Patterson, 1926; Hales, 1958; Stewart *et al.*, 1953; Gotshalk, Tessmer and Smith, 1940; Chaudry *et al.*, 1960; Friedrich and Renaud, 1960; Hoggins and Thornton, 1958). In one case (Bernstein, 1929) the lesion was pulsatile. The degree of pigmentation may vary both in the primary tumour and in the secondary deposits (Patterson, 1926; Schoolman and Anderson, 1950; Mason and Friedmann, 1955; Friedmann, 1958), and some cases reported in the literature had flat oral pigmentation for up to 20 years before vertical growth developed. However, Baxter (1939) and Chaudhry *et al.* (1960) state that only about one-third or less of patients are known to have pre-existing oral pigmentation; I think this is probably an underestimate.

Allen and Spitz (1953) state that only half the mucosal melanomas are pigmented. According to Baxter (1939) the depth of pigmentation has no relationship to the malignancy of the tumour. The five cases seen at the

Melanoma Clinic were almost all dark brown or black, but there were small amelanotic areas of growth. Mulligan (1949) observed in dogs that the more anaplastic lesions had little pigment. In the patients reported by Hayton-Williams (1962) a flat pigmented area, which had been observed for nine years, became pigmented at first and this was followed in six months by increasing pigmentation.

The nodularity of the surface is often mentioned; it has also been described in buccal malignant melanoma in the dog (Povar and Povar, 1950). In spite of the bleeding and even the size of the growth, it seems to cause little inconvenience to the patient (Bernstein, 1929), and it is rarely painful (New and Hansel, 1921; Moore and Martin, 1955). The explanation for the lack of disturbance may be the negligible induration caused by the tumour and the absence of infection associated with it. The lack of sclerosis is typical of cutaneous melanoma and its metastasis (p. 81).

The growth may reach a considerable size before the adjacent bones are involved (Fig. 12.1) (Alsup, 1950). Hoggins and Thornton's (1958) case is somewhat exceptional in this regard as there was extensive bone involvement, but the tumour was growing very rapidly. Considerable bone involvement at an early stage suggests that the lesion is metastatic (Ringertz, 1938; de Cholnoky, 1941; Bluestone, 1953).

The two phases of growth (horizontal and vertical) may overlap considerably and the graduation between actively expanding tumour and flat pigmented patches is often imprecise. The rate of growth is also capricious; some lesions follow a consistent and rapid course to death (Stewart et al., 1953; Hoggins and Thornton, 1958), other patients have a long drawn-out history of flat pigmentation before rapid growth supervenes, and when such a growth does occur, it may be very rapidly fatal (Hayton-Williams, 1962) or continue to be locally progressive with little sign of extensive spread (Patterson, 1926; Chaudhry et al., 1958; Chaudhry et al., 1960).

The first metastases are usually found in the cervical lymph nodes (de Cholnoky, 1941; Sir-sat, 1953). The enlarged nodes are usually painless (as in two of my cases); however, Seldin et al. (1958) observed the unusual features of marked tenderness in the enlarged nodes.

Sooner or later the disease usually becomes widely disseminated and, although any organ or tissue may harbour metastases (Shockett and Dembrow, 1963; Milton, 1952), those first detected are in the lungs (Bernstein, 1929; Chaudhry et al., 1958).

NOSE

The phase of slowly spreading pigmentation seen so frequently in oral malignant melanoma has not been observed in nasal lesions. However, benign pigmented areas in the nose are very uncommon. Mason and Friedmann (1955) saw eight benign pigmented lesions in the nose, and Ravid and Esteves (1960) reported one juvenile melanoma. Whether such lesions are precursors of nasal malignant melanoma is problematical because the usual history is one of polyps, which may not be pigmented. Once the melanoma has become apparent, the history is of frequent epistaxis, a nasal obstruction, the duration of symptoms as a rule being measured in months (Schoolman and Anderson, 1950; Collins, 1930; Ringertz, 1938; Grace, 1947; Alsup, 1950; Alexander, 1954; Mason and Friedmann, 1955; Ravid and Esteves, 1960; Shafer, Hine and Levy, 1963). The melanoma is frequently pigmented, but the depth of pigmentation may vary and the local recurrence may be free of pigmentation (Mason and Friedmann, 1955; Ringertz, 1938). As in the mouth, the lesions do not appear to involve the bone at early stages and pain is a rare symptom (Ringertz, 1938). The melanoma may present at the vestibule and occasionally involve the skin secondarily (Shafer et al., 1963). The lymph nodes of the neck are usually the first site of metastases, and generalised metastases frequently take years to develop.

Diagnosis

The diagnosis of both oral and nasal malignant melanoma can only be established by biopsy. Pigmentation in the mouth in

Addison's disease and Peutz–Jaeger's syndrome is static relative to that due to melanoma, which is progressive. In addition, patients will often have other features suggesting the correct diagnosis. Accidental tattooing on the gum produced by amalgam or carborundum wheel is also static (Seldin et al., 1958; Dwight, Weathers and Fine, 1974). Pigmentation of the gingivae from bismuth or lead is characteristic in its situation close to the teeth, and the colour is grey or blue, rather than black (Abrahams, 1954). A submucosal haemangioma may resemble a melanoma except that it is rare on the palate, is compressible and tends to remain stationary for years. Close inspection shows a haemangioma to be submucosal rather than of the mucosa and finally it has no surrounding discolouration. Another form of submucosal pigmentation is the blue naevus in which the collection of darkly pigmented melanocytes may look alarming but the healthy mucosa covering them and the long history without growth should suggest the diagnosis.

Greene et al. (1954) suggested three criteria for diagnosis:

1. The cellular characteristics may be those of a malignant melanoma.
2. Areas of junctional activity must be demonstrated.
3. No other primary can be found.

However, they and Chaudhry et al. (1958) point out that junctional activity may be hard to demonstrate in an ulcerating lesion as it is in some cutaneous melanomas.

The presence of pigment does not automatically diagnose malignant melanoma, as haemosiderin can cause a deep pigmentation (Haymann, 1888; Ringertz, 1938; Ravid and Esteves, 1960). Pigmentation due to both iron and melanin may coexist in the same tumour.

The clinical history combined with the histological features 'sarcomatous' or 'carcinomatous' should supply the diagnosis, even in the absence of deep pigmentation (Willis, 1948; Allen, 1949; Allen and Spitz, 1953; Friedmann, 1958; Sisson, Johnson and Amiri, 1963).

Multicentric origin

There have been many suggestions that these lesions arise from multicentric foci (Allen and Spitz, 1953; Friedrich and Renaud, 1960; Conley and Pack, 1963). Hayton-Williams (1962) referred to the danger of 'skip' lesions in the treatment of this disease. In three cases seen at the Melanoma Clinic, the lesions could have been of multicentric origin, because the growth of tumour was patchy with healthy mucosa between. The pigmentation of the mucosa could have been a reflection of a general instability which sooner or later becomes aggressively malignant. Certainly the possibility of multicentricity of the tumour should be remembered during the follow-up of patients after the first treatment.

Treatment

The prophylactic excision of pigmented patches in the mouth of dark-skinned people would not be feasible as oral pigmentation is frequent. The problem is different with Caucasians. If the pigmentation is spreading in the mouth, especially on the palate, the need for excision is urgent. If the theories of multicentric origin and mucosal instability mentioned above are valid, careful follow-up examinations are essential.

In nasal lesions, the preliminary pigmentation is not so likely to be detected, but the same careful follow-up after excision is obligatory.

The best method of treating oral malignant melanoma is to establish the diagnosis by biopsy and follow this by diathermy curettage down to the healthy underlying tissues. The diathermy should be set on coagulation and no cutting current used because these lesions are vascular and, with the bloodless field produced in this way, the demarcation between the tumour and the underlying tissues can be easily demonstrated. The wound is left to granulate and heal by secondary intention, which it does with remarkable speed. The postoperative pain is controlled by analgesics for the first few days, but usually within a week frequent mouthwashes are all that is required to maintain healthy granulations and the patient is virtually pain-free. Meticulous follow-up examination at monthly intervals is essential for two years, not to detect recurrence in the treated area, but because of the risk of a second primary developing. Any subsequent tumour is treated by curettage if it is large; if it is less than 0·5 cm diameter, it can usually be destroyed with an intralesional injection of 15 mg thiotepa in 0·5 ml water. The use of diathermy in one form or another has been mentioned by several authors (New and Hansel, 1921; Patterson, 1926; Mason and Friedmann, 1955; Gignoux et al., 1959; Kragh and Erich, 1960; Conley and Pack, 1963; Chaudhry et al., 1958).

The management of the draining lymph nodes is still a subject of debate. If the primary tumour is flat, I think prophylactic lymph node resection is unnecessary, while if an otherwise young and healthy person has a raised and nodular lesion, prophylactic lymph node resection of the suprahymoid region is probably desirable.

I think radiotherapy is not the treatment of choice because it is often ineffective in controlling the primary growth. In one of my cases it caused bone necrosis which allowed the tumour access to the hard palate. Even massive primary melanoma will not penetrate a healthy periosteum (Adair, 1936; Ringertz, 1938; Grace, 1947; Stewart, 1951; Chaudhry et al., 1958; Friedmann, 1958; Conley and Pack, 1963; Rubenfield, 1962; Tweedie, 1933; Schoolman and Anderson, 1950; Seldin et al., 1958; Hayton-Williams, 1962; Madigan,1962).

The same principles apply to nasal malignant melanoma. Wide diathermy excision is usually recommended (Tweedie, 1933; Capps and Williams, 1950; Morris and Horn, 1951). Tweedie (1933) also noticed that the pigmented tumours stripped off the underlying bone easily (as in the mouth). Prophylactic excision of lymph nodes is probably not justified, as local recurrence is extremely frequent and generalised dissemination occurs in the great majority of patients sooner or later, no matter what treatment is given. However, Kragh and Erich (1960) have recommended removal of lymph nodes (their figures show some improvement on many series).

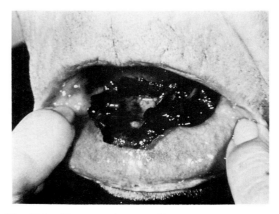

Fig. 12.1 Shows a primary malignant melanoma of the floor of the mouth in a 71-year-old man who had first observed oral pigmentation six years before this picture was taken. The lesion had grown slowly throughout this time, but it had remained painless and had caused little if any change in either his speech or his ability to swallow. He sought treatment because the lesion started to bleed. The tumour did not involve the mandible, and following diathermy curettage the wound healed.

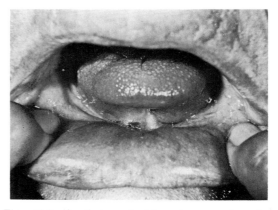

Fig. 12.2 A photograph taken two months after treatment. Apart from one small area of recurrent tumour, also dealt with by diathermy, the patient remained well for at least three years when he was lost to follow-up.

Conclusion

Melanoma arising in the mucosa of the nose or mouth is a dangerous disease, and the danger is greatly increased when the tumour changes from horizontal to vertical growth. Brown flat pigmentation of the oro-nasal mucosa should be removed by diathermy curettage before vertical growth has developed. However, even after extensive vertical growth has become established, diathermy curettage will rid the patient of the primary tumour. The correct method of treatment for sites of potential spread is still undecided, but if the primary lesion shows marked vertical growth, prophylactic lymph node clearance is probably justified in young and fit patients. However, meticulous follow-up after initial surgery is essential because:

1. The primary tumour may be multicentric and new primary lesions therefore appear at any time.

2. Careful study of the pattern of the disease may develop to solve the riddle of correct treatment.

REFERENCES

Abrahams, A. (1954) *French's Index of Differential Diagnosis*, ed. Douthwaite, A. H. 7th edition, p. 632. Bristol: Wright.

Adair, F. E. (1936) Treatment of melanoma; report of four hundred cases. *Surgery, Gynecology and Obstetrics*, **62**, 406.

Alexander, F. W. (1954) Malignant melanoma of nasal septum. *Laryngoscope*, **64**, 123.

Allen, A. C. (1949) Reorientation on histogenesis and clinical significance of cutaneous naevi and melanomas. *Cancer*, **2**, 28.

Allen, A. C. & Spitz, S. (1953) Malignant melanoma; a clinicopathology analysis of the criteria for diagnosis and prognosis. *Cancer*, **6**, 1.

Alsup, W. B. (1950) Malignant melanoma of nasal cavity; review of American literature and report of case. *North Carolina Medical Journal*, **11**, 76.

Baxter, H. (1939) Malignant melanoma in the coloured races: Report of case originating in the mouth. *Canadian Medical Association Journal*, **41**, 350.

Bernstein, J. (1929) Melano-carcinoma of the hard palate. *The Journal of Laryngology and Otology*, **44**, 328.

Bluestone, L. I. (1953) Malignant melanoma metastatic to the mandible; report of a case. *Oral Surgery, Oral Medicine and Oral Pathology*, **6**, 237.

Capps, F. C. W. & Williams, I. G. (1950) Discussion on malignant diseases of the nasal cavity and sinuses. *Proceedings of the Royal Society of Medicine*, **43**, 665.

Charalambidis, P. H. & Patterson, W. B. (1962) A clinical study of 250 patients with malignant melanoma. *Surgery, Gynecology and Obstetrics*, **115**, 333.

Chaudhry, A. P., Gorlin, R. J. & Reynolds, D. H. (1960) Sialolithiasis of a minor salivary gland. *Oral Surgery, Oral Medicine and Oral Pathology*, **13**, 578.

Chaudhry, A. P., Hampel, A., & Gorlin, R. J. (1958) Primary malignant melanoma of the oral cavity; a review of 105 cases. *Cancer*, **11**, 923.

Collins, E. G. (1930) A case of melanoma of the nose. *Journal of Laryngology and Otology*, **45**, 691.

Conley, J. J. & Pack, G. T. (1963) Melanoma of the head and neck. *Surgery, Gynecology and Obstetrics*, **116**, 15.

Cotchin, E. (1955) Melanotic tumours of dogs. *Journal of Comparative Pathology and Therapeutics*, **65**, 115.

Daland, E. M. (1959) Malignant melanoma; personal experience with 170 cases. *The New England Journal of Medicine*, **260**, 453.

de Cholnoky, T. (1941) Malignant melanoma; a clinical study of one hundred and seventeen cases. *Annals of Surgery*, **113**, 392.

Dwight, R., Weathers, D. D. S. & Fine, R. M. (1974) Amalgam tattoo of oral mucosa. *Archives of Dermatology*, **110**, 727.

Friedmann, I. (1958) *Cancer*, ed. Raven, R. W. Vol. 2, p. 575. London: Butterworth.

Friedrich, E. G. & Renaud, O. V. (1960) Primary malignant melanoma of the oral cavity: report of case. *Journal of Oral Surgery, Anesthesia and Hospital Dental Service*, **18**, 336.

Gignoux, M., Papillon, J., Caillard, J., *et al.* (1959) Apropos of an observation on a melanic tumour of nasal fossa. *Annals of Otology, Rhinology and Laryngology*, **76**, 1120.

Gotshalk, H. C., Tessmer, C. F. & Smith, J. W. (1940) Malignant melanoma of palate. *Archives of Pathology*, **30**, 762.

Grace, C. C. (1947) Malignant melanoma of nasal mucosa. *Archives of Otolaryngology*, **46**, 195.

Greene, G. W., Haynes, J. W., Dozier, M., *et al.* (1954) Primary malignant melanoma of the oral mucosa. *Oral Surgery, Oral Medicine and Oral Pathology*, **6**, 1435.

Hales, W. B. (1958) Malignant melanoma of the hard and soft palate. *Proceedings of the Royal Society of Medicine*, **51**, 698.

Hart, V. K. (1943) Some rhinolaryngological tumors of unusual clinical interest; small series presenting infrequent character, difficulty in management, or both. *North Carolina Medical Journal*, **4**, 497.

Haymann (1888) Quoted by Ringertz, N. (1938) Pathology of malignant melanoma arising in nasal and paranasal cavities and maxilla. *Acta oto-laryngologica*, Supp., **27**, 1.

Hayton-Williams, D. S. (1962) A case of intra-oral melanoma: innocence to malignancy. *Proceedings of the Royal Society of Medicine*, **55**, 485.

Hewer, T. F. (1935) Malignant melanoma in coloured races: the role of trauma in its causation. *Journal of Pathology and Bacteriology*, **41**, 473.

Hoggins, G. S. & Thornton, K. R. (1958) Melanoma of the hard palate. *Proceedings of the Royal Society of Medicine*, **51**, 696.

Kragh, L. V. & Erich, J. B. (1960) Malignant melanomas of the head and neck. *Annals of Surgery*, **151**, 91.

Madigan, J. P. (1962) Symposium on oxygen barotherapy: a preliminary clinical report concerning oxygen barotherapy and megavoltage radiotherapy. *Journal of the College of Radiologists of Australasia*, **6**, 94.

Mason, M. & Friedmann, I. (1955) Melanoma of the nose and ear. *Journal of Laryngology and Otology*, **69**, 98.

Milton, G. W. (1952) Occurrence of secondary malignant disease in spleen. *Medical Journal of Australia*, **2**, 736.

Milton, G. W. & Lane Brown, M. M. (1965) Malignant melanoma of the nose and mouth. *British Journal of Surgery*, **52**, 484.

Moore, E. S. & Martin, H. (1955) Melanoma of the upper respiratory tract and oral cavity. *Cancer*, **8**, 1167.

Morey, G. (1952) A case of nasal melanoma. *Journal of Laryngology and Otology*, **66**, 191.

Morris, G. C., Jr, & Horn, R. C., Jr (1951) Malignant melanoma in the negro; review of the literature and report of nine cases. *Surgery*, **29**, 223.

Mulligan, R. M. (1949) Neoplastic diseases of dogs; I. Neoplasms of melanin-forming cells. *American Journal of Pathology*, **25**, 339.

New, G. B. & Hansel, F. K. (1921) Melano-epithelioma of the palate. *Journal of the American Medical Association*, **77**, 19.

Pack, G. T., Gerber, D. M. & Scharnagel, I. M. (1952) End results in the treatment of malignant melanoma; a report of 1190 cases. *Annals of Surgery*, **136**, 905.

Patterson, N. (1926) Clinical record, melanoma of the hard palate. *Journal of Laryngology and Otology*, **41**, 32.

Povar, M. L. & Povar, R. (1950) Malignant melanoma of the oral mucosa in a dog. *Journal of the American Veterinary Medical Association*, **117**, 223.

Prinz, H. (1932) Pigmentations of the oral mucous membrane. *Dental Cosmos*, **74**, 554.

Ravid, J. M. & Esteves, J. A. (1960) Malignant melanoma of the nose and paranasal sinuses and juvenile melanoma of the nose. *Archives of Otolaryngology*, **72**, 431.

Ringertz, N. (1938) Pathology of malignant tumours arising in nasal and paranasal cavities and maxilla. *Acta oto-laryngologica*, Supp., **27**, 1.

Rubenfield, S. (1962) Melanoma of the nasal air passages. *Jewish Memorial Hospital Bulletin*, **6**, 119.

Schoolman, J. G. & Anderson, H. W. (1950) Malignant melanoma of the nose and sinuses. *Annals of Otology, Rhinology and Laryngology*, **59**, 124.

Seldin, H. M., Seldin, S. D., Rakower, W., et al. (1958) Malignant melanoma; report of a case. *Oral Surgery, Oral Medicine and Oral Pathology*, **11**, 1110.

Shafer, W. G., Hine, M. K. & Levy, B. M. (1963) *A Textbook of Oral Pathology*. 2nd edition, p. 79. Philadelphia: Saunders.

Shockett, E. & Dembrow, V. D. (1963) Splenic metastases from a melanoma of the nasal mucosa; the only thoraco-abdominal manifestation. *American Journal of Surgery*, **106**, 949.

Sirsat, M. V. (1953) Malignant melanoma of the mouth. *Indian Journal of Medical Research*, **41**, 119.

Sisson, G. A., Johnson, N. E. & Amiri, C. S. (1963) Cancer of the maxillary sinus. Clinical classification and management. *Annals of Otology, Rhinology and Laryngology*, **72**, 1050.

Smuts, P. A. (1939) Melanotic sarcoma of nasal septum. *South African Medical Journal*, **13**, 287.

Stewart, D. E., Hay, L. J. & Varco, R. L. (1953) Malignant melanomas: 92 cases treated at the University of Minnestoa Hospital since January 1, 1932. *Surgery, Gynecology and Obstetrics*, section: *International Abstracts of Surgery*, **97**, 209.

Stewart, T. S. (1951) Nasal malignant melanoma. *Journal of Laryngology and Otology*, **65**, 560.

Tweedie, A. R. (1933) Clinical Records: a case of melanotic sarcoma of the nose. *Journal of Laryngology and Otology*, **48**, 417.

Villa, V. G. & Laico, J. E. (1961) Intradermal nevus in the oral cavity evidently developing into a primary melanoma: Report of case. *Journal of Oral Surgery, Anesthesia and Hospital Dental Service*, **19**, 329.

Willis, R. A. (1948) *Pathology of Tumours*. London: Butterworth.

13. The Care of the Melanoma Patient and the Care of the Dying

The surgeon responsible for the care of patients suffering from malignant melanoma will soon find that one of the most difficult aspects of the management is to maintain the delicate balance of mental rapport between himself and the patient and his family, which will help him, the surgeon, ease the patient's mental distress. The problem of managing the patient's emotional stress is not easily subjected to statistical evaluation because each interview is essentially a one-to-one encounter and it is more important to appreciate the anxiety of the patient sitting opposite you than to know what 85·5 per cent of patients think when discussing their problems. One of the arts of medicine in this situation resembles the art of literature and consists of understanding human feelings.

Generally speaking, the thoughts of the patient suffering from malignant melanoma will pass through several stages. The first is when he realises that he has a disease which could be malignant. Prior to this he may be ignorant that the black spot has any sinister significance. The second stage evolves when the patient believes the disease *is* malignant. At this stage the condition is considered curable by the patient, his relatives and his doctor. The third stage in the patient's mental adjustment to his disease develops when it becomes increasingly obvious, first to the doctor and later to the patient and his relatives, that the disease is no longer curable. The last stage is that of the dying patient who is being destroyed by the disease (Milton, 1972 and 1973a).

Although the thoughts of a patient with melanoma will generally pass through the above stages, there are, of course, as many exceptions as there are methods of coping with bad news. For example, some patients may completely arrest their mental processes and block out any possibility of considering they may have a fatal disease; this process may be actively encouraged by the patient's medical advisors. As the disease advances the possibility of denying the approaching death becomes increasingly difficult for both the patient and his doctor. In any case an approaching death which can no longer be disregarded will affect a group of people. (I am only concerned here with the dying adult because melanoma in childhood is so rare; I will not extend this discussion into the emotional care of the dying child.) The centre of the group is the victim and the first circle around him is his immediate relatives, his parents and his dependants. In later stages there is a second ring about the sick patient which consists of those who are professionally connected with the patient, that is doctors, nurses, ministers, lawyers, etc. Outside this again are the workmates, employers or employees. Friends or casual acquaintances make up the next circle around the seriously ill. Finally, for public figures, comes the indifferent or curious general public.

The patient enters the first stage of adjusting to his disease in one of two ways. First, the patient who is ignorant of any possibility of malignancy and goes to his doctor with the idea that he has a trivial 'mole' may be suddenly confronted with the possibility of dying of cancer. Many people regard the word 'cancer' as synonymous with a death sentence. The second method of entry into the first stage of mental adjustment to malignancy will be the patient who has had a variety of symptoms for weeks or months which have gradually aroused in him a fear that he may have a malignant disease.

The mode of entry into the first stage will have an effect on the patient's ability to cope with the facts of cancer. All of us in times of great distress need some minimal time to become mentally acclimatised to misfortune. The sudden death sentence to the patient unaware of the potential of his disease may quite distort his adjustment and lead to irrational fear and reactions. On the other hand, the patient with some inkling of his condition may possibly welcome an intelligent discussion as soon as he sees his doctor.

Stage one. The first reaction of most people when they realise they might have cancer is fear, and the fear is directed in several ways. There is a fear of dying and the unknown, a fear of being dead and of leaving loved ones and happy associations. The patient often dreads the treatment, even if successful. But in addition to these anxieties, the patient may also be very apprehensive in case he reveals himself to be a coward and he may try various deceptions to conceal his fear. One way in which this is done is for the patient to say, 'Of course, I am not a bit worried about myself, I have had a good life, but I am really concerned about my wife and children.' The repetition of this or similar phrases often leads one to suppose that 'The lady doth protest too much, methinks'. On the other hand a young man with a family may genuinely feel guilty at deserting his wife: 'What a mess I got you into, we should never have got married.'

As these dreads develop in the patient's mind, another feeling may arise—a suspicion that his doctor and family are not telling him the truth. The wonderful account in Othello of the devastating effects of jealousy shows how a fine handkerchief can be taken as concrete proof of bad news to a jealous man. The same trivial evidence may be taken as important proof of imminent death by a patient suspicious that he is being deceived by his doctor and family. Once the patient's suspicions are aroused every word said by the surgeon, family doctor, resident medical officers, ward sisters, even hospital porters, is likely to be analysed

to ascertain if the remark contained a good or bad omen. In this way, the patient's mind builds a vicious circle of fear, doubt and suspicion; each emotion feeds on the others.

When the diagnosis has been established, the patient moves into *stage two* because his suspicions become more or less accepted fact; at this time another emotion will be grafted on to the previous ones. This can best be expressed as 'Why me?' In other words, as the diagnosis of malignancy becomes established the patient realises for the first time in his life that the dread word cancer is not something which affects other people. 'This time it's *me*'. This is a terrible blow to the patient and may require considerable adjustment because the natural response to the question 'Why me?' tends to be one of self-pity and resentment, which may be the next emotions felt by the sufferer. 'Why should I get this? I never did any harm to anybody, as have some people I know; I never have any luck.' The egocentricity shown by self-pity often leads the patient into being both irascible and unreasonable. 'They don't understand what I have to face.' 'You really don't care what happens to me.' These latter feelings tend to become more and more marked as stage two runs into *stage three* when the disease is evidently incurable. The egocentricity at this stage tends to augment a feeling of loneliness, which consists of both insulation and isolation from the community, and the loneliness often alternates with resentment and bitterness.

An understanding of the loneliness felt by a person approaching death is so crucial to his care that it is necessary to consider it in a little detail. The feeling of loneliness of the dying patient has been expressed well by many great writers. Chaucer in 'The Knight's Tale' has the dying Arcite say:

What is the world? What asken man to have?
Now with his love, now in his colde grave,
Alone withouten any company.

Dr Johnson in an essay in *The Idler* wrote 'Every inhabitant of the earth must walk downward to the grave alone and unregarded, without any partner of his joy or grief, without any interested witness of his misfortunate or success.'

The sudden isolation of the patient with cancer is well expressed by Solzhenitsyn in *Cancer Ward*. The successful family man Pavel Rusanov has been taken to Ward 13 because of a rapidly growing tumour in his neck. After his wife and son have left the hospital Rusanov's thoughts turn to his family life '... the harmonious, exemplary Rusanov family, their well-adjusted way of life and their immaculate apartment, in the space of a few days all this had been cut off from him. It was now on the *other* side of his tumour. They were alive and would go on living whatever happened to their father. However much they worry, fuss or weep, the tumour was growing like a wall behind him and on his side of it he was *alone*.' (This latter emphasis is my own.)

The fears of death will be discussed below in more detail but as the patient is in stage three and moving towards the inevitable death, his distress may be greatly augmented by a tantalising process where the melanoma appears to be cured and he has triumphed over the effects of surgery. He no sooner feels himself on the mend when the disease recurs and his hopes are dashed. It is likely in these periods of recurrent disease that the patient will develop symptoms of an anxiety neurosis, particularly headaches. As death becomes inevitable two more fears begin to play on the patient's mind. One is a fear of pain and the other the fear of indignity.

The problem of managing pain in advanced malignant melanoma has been dealt with elsewhere (p. 93), but the fear of loss of dignity lurks in the patient's mind. This is because it is unlikely, in our society, that he will have seen much of death except possibly an elderly relative whose gradual deterioration in advanced age he has viewed with distaste. The patient thinks that this process of disintegration is produced by malignancy rather than senility. Patients are nearly always aware of whispered conversations held supposedly out of earshot by nurses, medical students, or even the doctor and the patient's family. The idea of being converted into a 'thing' may have been implanted in the patient's mind when on a previous hospital admission he may have seen terminal patients almost ignored by nurses, doctors and visitors. A ward sister, while standing at the end of the bed of a dying patient, may have issued a staccato directive to a junior nurse. 'This patient must be turned two hourly, nurse', and move on without a backward glance. The senior surgeon comes to the end of such a patient's bed, 'Nothing to do here, Sister' and hurries on. Not a reassuring sight for one anticipating the ordeal himself. It is hardly surprising that with all these thoughts developing in his mind the patient approaching death is likely to become severely depressed.

Before discussing the management of the patient and his family during these different stages of mental adjustment, it is necessary to take a short look at the doctor's own reaction to malignant disease and death. All of us in the medical profession at one time or another are concerned with a patient with cancer and most of us are capable of dealing with them in a kindly but detached way. One of the techniques that the doctor uses to cope with patients with malignant disease is, of course, a protective denial for himself. The patient has a cancer while he, the doctor, is healthy and is unlikely to get it in the future. However, when the doctor is faced with death as distinct from the disease, he knows that he will himself die and thus finds it more difficult to cope with a dying patient. John Hinton (1967) quotes the case of a woman who knew she was going to die and wanted an opportunity to talk to the surgeon who originally treated her. The surgeon was unable to see the patient because of the pressure of work, but 'he also indicated that he was not sorry to have grounds to avoid such an interview'. The surgeon approaching a dying patient is also confronted by his own failure to cure the disease.

The difficulties in managing a cancer patient who is reaching the terminal stages stems partly from the hopelessness of any attempt at cure and partly from the attending staff's difficulty of coping with their own fear of death. I have seen surgeons, even of great eminence, who cannot face the dying, and needless to say this inability on the part of the eminent to cope with the dying has extensive repercussions. Not only does the family feel disappointed, even betrayed, but the junior staff in training soon learn that the 'great man' abandons an incurable patient and may put this into practice in their own working life.

It should be apparent from what has been said above that the management of a dying patient with malignant melanoma begins at the first encounter between the doctor and the patient and his family. This is important because it is never easy to communicate effectively and it may be virtually impossible to do so when the patient has death staring him in the face. The trust, friendship and understanding needed for effective communication has to be established from the first interview so that if a crisis develops and death becomes imminent, there is a firm foundation for effective rapport.

If the family doctor suspects that he is referring a patient with malignant melanoma to a surgeon it is desirable to have both the patient and their next of kin attend the consultation together. There are two reasons for this. Firstly the situation of speaking once to the patient and separately to the next of kin is certain to increase the patient's suspicion that the truth is too horrible for him to be told. The inevitable consequence of these thoughts is to increase the patient's feeling of isolation. The very people he wishes to trust the most, his wife and his doctor, are the ones who whisper behind his back. The second reason for having patient and relative interviewed together is that the fear of mutilation can often be partly alleviated by the wife assuring the husband (if he is the patient) that it will not distress her. In addition if the condition is suspected of being malignant it is not infrequent for the patient to end up supporting his wife at the first interview and the bond of a successful marriage gives great strength at this time.

During the initial interview it is most important that the surgeon explains to the patient in easily understood language the nature of the patient's disease. However, he must bear in mind that the patient may need time to become acclimatised to misfortune. It is also vital that he does not prevaricate by changing his decision, as this tends to be given distorted significance in a suspicious mind. Hence, if the patient has what appears clinically to be a malignant melanoma, the most humane course of action is to explain that this may be a malignant condition, that on the present indications it is curable, however, the final verdict of malignancy depends on the examination of the tissue. Therefore, an initial biopsy gives the patient an opportunity to adjust to his condition. If the clinician is very experienced in melanoma and can be virtually certain on clinical grounds that it is malignant, then other means of allowing the patient time to adjust to the possibility of cancer are easy to find, e.g. order a chest X-ray and request another interview.

Although a carefully given verbal explanation about his disease is of great help to the patient, we have found in the Melanoma Clinic that it helps the patient and his family to have a simply worded written document to take home and read at leisure. The written word can be discussed by the patient and his family in the security of his home and allows them time to 'digest' the new information important to them (Ch. 3, p. 44).

At the second interview the proposed course of treatment is discussed together with means of diagnosis (e.g. frozen section). In the early interviews it is unnecessary to talk of death and the doctor should concentrate solely on the ways and means of dealing with the disease. The fear of mutilation must be faced and the morbidity from block dissections, discussed elsewhere in this book, explained to the patient and his wife. The patient should also be asked if he has any questions, which are promptly answered truthfully but accentuating the favourable features. By these means the patient's initial suspicions can be reduced.

Immediately after the initial operation if glands have been dissected and found to be negative and the prognosis appears favourable, the patient and his relatives are told of the result of the operation and hopeful features are stressed. Again the patient and family are asked if they have any questions. Never under any circumstances at this point say to the wife, 'Can I see you outside for a minute please?'

Occasionally a well-meaning relative will say, 'Please don't tell him if it's malignant, I'm sure he would go to pieces.' When this happens I usually try to persuade the relatives that attempts at deception are bound to fail because the treatment and the relatives' own behaviour will imply the truth to any intelligent person. If deception is attempted and fails the patient will feel let down and isolated, so the wiser course is to have a frank and kindly conference with the relatives and the patient. Few families have objected to this and none, so far as I am aware, have regretted it afterwards.

If the disease starts to recur months or even years later, then it is well to face the facts of cancer in a realistic way. The great majority of patients are able to adjust to the realities of cancer better than to a fool's paradise they know to be false. Certainly after the original discussions the patient may cope with his disease by a process of denial; it would be un-likely for him to do anything else considering how both as individuals and as groups we deny death.

The denial is exhibited by a variety of beha-vioural patterns. The patient may accept that the doctor has told him the truth as the doctor sees it but will be adamant that his doctor is wrong. It is neither necessary nor humane to break down this form of denial. Secondly, the patient may demonstrate considerable bon-homie and the young doctor may be amazed at, say, Mr Smith, who is facing up to his situa-tion incredibly well. Smith is jocular, cheerful and will make fun at various methods of treatment which may be used. His attendances at clinic may be accompanied by much giggling from the nurses as he chats amicably to all and sundry. The old hands will recognise this spurious jocularity as a denial mechanism which may suddenly break down, and if it does, the patient's appearance and attitude will alter overnight from one of excessive good cheer to one of indifference and lethargy, and the patient will probably die within a month from what may be described as a psychological death (Milton, 1973b). The third defence mechan-ism is for the patient to accept the diagnosis but reject the consequences. Such a patient may be deprived of all his fortune by any well-meaning quack or even absolute charlatan who claims to cure cancer. Such patients may say, 'Well the cure can't do me any harm and who knows it may do some good; it is worth a try' (Milton, 1975).

The adult manner of coping with inevitable and imminent distress or death is to accept the situation, make what personal or family arrangements are feasible and not to dwell any more than can be helped on the terrors of the adjacent future. It is surprising how many people are able to adjust to their fate in this way and enjoy their remaining life provided they are properly cared for.

The essence, then, of coping with cancer as far as the relationship between the doctor and his patient and family is concerned is one of humane honesty which begins at the first inter-view and continues to death. It is vital that the consultant who tends the patient initially does not abandon him once he feels cure is no longer possible, but retains sufficient interest to see the patient and talk with him even if he can do nothing more. However, beware of exces-sive pity because the patient is always on the verge of self-pity and lamentation from the senior specialist is likely to precipitate the patient into a trough of unhappiness. At all interviews stress positive and helpful ap-proaches rather than negative ones. Instead of 'nothing more can be done', talk of modern chemotherapy (p. 84), rare cases of spon-taneous remission or the efficacy of pain relief. It is sometimes helpful to talk of family affairs; I had one young farmer with advanced melanoma who discussed how his wife could manage their property until his sons were old enough to take over. This conversation helped both the wife and husband—the latter felt a sense of his own continuity through his child-ren.

The patient should always be treated as a sensible adult. The well-meaning ward sister who says, 'We are a little better today, aren't we?' as if she were talking to a five-year-old should be warned that few adults like being regarded as infantile.

Throughout the process of the care of these patients, the surgeon and all his staff work as a team with nurses, churchmen, social workers and the patient and his family. The leader of the team may vary from time to time, but suc-cessful management of the patient with a melanoma depends on each member of the team trusting each other, and in this way the mental anguish and loneliness of the uncured patient may be considerably alleviated. A modest achievement but one worth attaining.

REFERENCES

Hinton, J. (1967) *Dying*, p. 11. Harmondsworth, Middlesex: Penguin Books.
Milton, G. W. (1972) The care of the dying. *The Medical Journal of Australia*, **2,** 177.
Milton, G. W. (1973a) Thoughts in mind of a person with cancer. *British Medical Journal*, iv, 221.
Milton, G. W. (1973b) Self-willed death or the bone-pointing syndrome. *Lancet*, i, 1435.
Milton, G. W. (1975) The cure of cancer. *Modern Medicine of Australia*, **18,** 8.

Index